LIGHT UP YOUR BLUES

Understanding and Overcoming Seasonal Affective Disorders

by:
Robert N. Moreines, M.D.
and
Patricia L. McGuire, M.D.

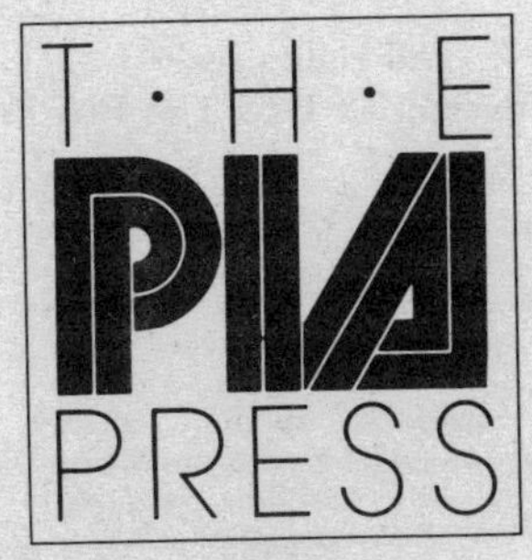

This book is not intended to replace personal medical care and supervision; there is no substitute for the experience and information that a doctor can provide. Rather, it is our hope that this book will provide additional information to help people understand the proper use of medication in biopsychiatry.

Proper medical care should always be tailored to the individual patient. If you read something in this book that seems to conflict with your doctor's instructions, contact your doctor. Your doctor may have medically sound reasons for prescribing medication in a manner that may differ from the information presented in this book.

Also note that this book may not contain every drug or brand of drug currently prescribed in the treatment of Seasonal Affective Disorder.

If you have any questions about any medicine or treatment in this book, consult your doctor or pharmacist.

In addition, the patient names and cases used do not represent actual people, but are composite cases drawn from several sources.

For information address:
Psychiatric Institutes of America,
part of the National Medical Enterprises Specialty Hospital Group.
1010 Wisconsin Ave. NW
Washington, D.C. 20007

CONTENTS

DEDICATION

To my wife, Susan, and my son, Jared.

—Robert N. Moreines, M.D.

To the scholars and mentors that have changed the course of my life: John F. McGuire, M.D.; Paul R. McHugh, M.D.; Andrew E. Slaby, M.D., Ph.D., M.P.H.; A. L. Carter Pottash, M.D.; and Natalie Shainess, M.D.

—Patricia L. McGuire, M.D.

ACKNOWLEDGEMENTS

We are especially grateful to Ron Schaumburg, whose outstanding talents contributed greatly to the creation of this book.

In addition, we would like to thank our colleagues at Fair Oaks Hospital and to our patients, who have shown us that it is indeed possible to overcome Seasonal Affective Disorders.

LIGHT UP YOUR BLUES

Understanding and Overcoming Seasonal Affective Disorders

by:
Robert N. Moreines, M.D.
and
Patricia L. McGuire, M.D.

Chapter 1

THE PATIENT WITH SEASONAL AFFECTIVE DISORDER

During much of the year, Jenny was a happy, healthy, energetic woman. She loved her family and her friends, doted on her two daughters, and put in long hours as an executive secretary for a New Jersey insurance firm. Jenny, a dark-haired woman in her mid-thirties, described herself as a "nonstop talker and a real live wire" who loved summertime activities: water-skiing, hiking, and bicycling.

But in a very real sense, Jenny* lived under a cloud. As the frolics of summer ended and her children returned to school, she would feel a twinge of anxiety, bordering on fear, that something inside her was about to change. When the leaves began to change colors in October, Jenny experienced a nameless sense of dread. She noticed that it became increasingly difficult to get out of bed in the morning. As time went on, her energy continued to flag; soon she began to leave work a little earlier each day, exhausted by the same daily routine that she had managed so well just a few months earlier.

Her eating habits began to change, too; she felt mysterious

---

*All patient names have been changed and identities disguised to protect privacy.

cravings for candies and pastries, foods she seldom ate during the summer. Jenny rationalized her new diet as an attempt to restore her dwindling reserves of energy. However, she failed to gain the energy she sought; she did, however, gain some extra pounds.

By the time Thanksgiving arrived, Jenny had turned into the mirror image of her "summer self"—moody, lethargic, quick to snap at her daughters or her husband, Walter. She became more and more withdrawn from family activities. Each night she went to bed a little earlier, until finally she was sleeping between ten and twelve hours a night.

With the onset of winter, Walter found himself shouldering virtually the entire burden of planning and carrying out the Christmas rituals, including shopping, wrapping gifts, and entertaining friends and relatives. Most of the time Jenny was upstairs in the bedroom, trying to "catch up on her sleep." Despite the extra hours in bed, she never felt completely rested.

The girls made up excuses to explain their mother's odd behavior to visitors. "Mom hates winter," they would say. "She's like a bear—she hibernates." Each year, as the pattern began to reassert itself, Walter grew increasingly resentful of what he assumed was Jenny's poor attitude and her lack of concern for herself—and for him. He found himself wondering if their marriage would survive another winter of such discontent.

One day Walter spotted Jenny sitting glumly in her favorite chair and found himself unable to endure this picture of misery any longer. In a fit of pique he snapped, "Why don't you just pull yourself out of it?"

"I can't," she replied tearfully.

"Then you need help," he said bluntly, "and I can't give it to you."

His words struck home. The next day Jenny went to her family physician, who had treated her and her daughters for years, and described her situation. His diagnosis: mild depression. He wrote a prescription for a low-dosage antidepressant medication, gave her the name of a psychiatrist, and sent her on her way. She never made an appointment with the psychiatrist, and rationalized her choice by saying, "He'll tell me I feel this way because I hate my mother or something. And I know that's not the reason." She took her medicine faithfully, and noticed that it seemed to help a little, but she never completely felt her "old self."

Inevitably, however, spring arrived, and just as inevitably Jenny underwent a further transformation. As the days grew longer, her spirits rose and her old energy returned—"spring fever," she called it. She began to ride her bicycle again, to burn off the weight she had gained. Her sleep habits returned to her usual pattern of seven and a half hours per night. She threw herself into her work, accomplishing in a few hours what had taken her days to do in January. And she tossed the remainder of her antidepressant medication into the trash. Although Walter teasingly chided her about their growing phone bills, he was secretly happy that she was again chatting with distant friends. Her family, glad to have "the real Mom" back, quickly forgot about the darks days of winter and basked in the glow of Jenny's sunny disposition.

In the autumn of 1985, an event took place that changed Jenny's life and that of her family. It brought her to the attention of the medical staff at Fair Oaks Hospital in Summit, New Jersey.

One morning in late September, Jenny experienced some difficulty dragging herself out of bed. During breakfast she felt pangs of anxiety that she attributed to her dread of the coming winter. Somehow she managed to put those thoughts out of her head, at least temporarily.

Later that evening, while tidying up the house, she decided to update the family photo album, incorporating all the snapshots that had accumulated during the summer. She filled page after page with images of herself and the girls water-skiing, playing on the shore of their favorite lake, or performing stunts on their bicycles. In a nostalgic mood, Jenny turned back to the pictures taken during their hiking tour of Canada the summer before. There she was, backpack and all, waving happily as she trekked along the trail.

Then she began to turn the pages forward again. In doing so she gradually realized that pictures of herself grew increasingly rare. Those in which she did appear showed a woman whose face became more and more grim, and whose body grew less and less shapely. Come Christmas, Jenny had virtually faded away from the scene, until, as evidenced by the photos of her family's New Year's celebration, she had vanished entirely. Eventually, though, spring burgeoned and Jenny reappeared: Easter pictures showed her handsomely dressed and enjoying an egg hunt with her children. By summer she had once again become her old self: trim, vivacious, and happy.

To Jenny, the pages of the photo album were like a child's flip book—a mini-movie condensing months of action into a few seconds. She began to realize that she had repeated this seasonal pattern every year since she had graduated from college.

Just then Walter entered the room to show her an article he had spotted in the newspaper. The article described a newly identified form of mood disorder, one that could be triggered by the cycle of seasons and that caused such symptoms as fatigue, changes in appetite, and abnormal sleep patterns. Jenny listened intently. "Does that sound like anyone we know?" Walter asked. "Sure does," said Jenny. The treatment for the disorder, the article said, involved the use of light—pure bright light, administered in a carefully monitored program under the guidance of a physician—and for some people its effectiveness had proved nothing short of astounding.

The next day Jenny made an appointment at Fair Oaks Hospital, where she was asked to describe the history of her problem in detail. After this, she was given a thorough physical evaluation, which ruled out any medical reason for her condition, and a complete psychiatric assessment. When enough information had been collected, her condition was diagnosed: Jenny was found to suffer from Seasonal Affective Disorder, also known by the appropriate acronym SAD.

Fair Oaks Hospital, located in Summit, New Jersey, has a nationwide reputation as an institution on the leading edge of psychiatric medicine. Many patients come there after they have exhausted other options and still have not found the relief they seek. Because of Fair Oaks's special focus on biological psychiatry, the staff is alert to the needs of patients such as Jenny, whose depressive symptoms can be traced to a malfunction in the complex body systems responsible for controlling mood.

As psychiatrists we have seen hundreds of patients with depressions of all types. Our experience has helped us become particularly sensitive to the physiological origins of mental disorders, and to the unusual features encountered in affective (mood) disorders. By "physiological" we mean that certain organic malfunctions—for example, a thyroid gland that isn't producing enough vital hormones—can often lead to the symptoms associated with depression. The study of such glandular effects on the nervous system, called neuroendocrinology, is a relatively new but rapidly expanding medical discipline.

Our interest in SAD arose from our encounters with a special category of patients: those whose moods clearly demonstrated a seasonal pattern and who did not improve as much as expected after the use of antidepressant medications and other standard therapies. To help these patients, who are often described as "treatment-resistant," we needed to expand our outlook and explore the use of new and, to some minds, unusual therapeutic methods.

Working within a hospital setting as we do means that we have a number of important resources at our disposal. One such resource is the opportunity to interact with other psychiatric professionals at Fair Oaks and to exchange new knowledge about the causes and treatments of depression. We are particularly fortunate to know such talented and dedicated individuals as Dr. Robert Davies and Dr. Peter Mueller, whose insights into the relationship between seasonal fluctuations in mood and the therapeutic use of light have been particularly eye-opening.

In addition, the hospital places great emphasis on keeping abreast of new developments in the field, particularly in the use of medication. Thus we are obligated to keep ourselves constantly informed about the latest research into strategies for managing psychiatric illness, in order to take full advantage of the hope they offer.

At Fair Oaks we deal with depressed individuals primarily as inpatients and therefore have the opportunity to observe them closely over a period of time, using extensive neurodiagnostic evaluations to establish a valuable database. Our observations allow us to detect subtle changes in moods at very close range, and permit us to monitor the factors that trigger depressive symptoms as well as reactions to therapy. As physicians, we can't help but feel gratified when we see our patients improve— dramatically and rapidly—during light treatment.

Another factor comes into play at Fair Oaks: Our New Jersey location places us in a region of the country where winters are longer and darker than in, say, Florida. As a result of this geographic accident, we are more likely to encounter patients for whom SAD presents a problem than would otherwise be the case.

On a somewhat more personal level, another resource we can claim is the sense of excitement in finding ourselves alongside other investigators who are exploring a relatively uncharted field of psychiatry. Almost every day, new discoveries are made about the biological processes involved in mental disorders and the hitherto underestimated impact that our environment, including the climate, can have on mental health. Such discoveries are helping to answer some of the basic questions about SAD, including:

- What are the symptoms of SAD and how are these symptoms experienced by a patient?
- What type of person is at risk of developing this disorder?
- What does it mean to be a SAD patient? How does the illness affect people emotionally? What impact does it have on the ability to function at home, in the workplace, and in society as a whole?
- What are the practical issues confronting a physician who must first learn to recognize the illness and subsequently manage patients who suffer from it?

As coauthors, we bring a shared perspective—a kind of stereoscopic vision—to the subject of SAD and its impact. For that reason, and to make reading easier, the word "we" will be used throughout the narrative of the book to indicate our collective experiences with SAD at Fair Oaks. When necessary, however, distinctions will be made between the contributions of the two authors.

For example, while both of us see and treat depressed patients, Dr. Moreines focuses his interest primarily on the scientific and theoretical aspects of SAD, including the body mechanisms and the environmental factors involved. His interest in the disorder stems from his work on a team with Dr. Davies, who alerted him to the existence of SAD-like patterns in some of their patients. Dr. Moreines has a special interest in the decision process that leads to precise and correct diagnosis of mental disorders and in treatment for treatment-resistant patients; these interests, coupled with a treatment approach and innovative psychopharmacology that ties together the many different components of psychiatric therapy, made SAD a natural target for his study.

The other author, Dr. McGuire, has become Fair Oaks's

"resident expert" in managing SAD patients on a day-to-day basis. She traces her interest in the condition to the day she moved into a new office at the hospital and found that the previous occupant had left behind one of the light boxes used in SAD therapy. Having heard about the lights, and curious about their effects, she tried using them during a session with a patient whose depression had not been improving to the desired degree under a program of medication and psychotherapy. Much to her surprise, by the end of the hour-long session she detected improvement in the patient's mood.

Over the past several years, we have encountered many patients from a wide variety of backgrounds who have suffered from SAD to varying degrees. Among the cases on file are:

- Kathy, 41 years old. Winter was "the black hole" of her year. Her life in the summer was "terrific," she said, but she described herself as depressed and miserable throughout the dark months. Each year around Christmastime she would develop a syndrome of symptoms: fatigue, lethargy, aching muscles. "I slow down like a music box that needs winding," she remarked. The symptoms, which persisted until spring, caused a pervasive depression, crankiness, slower or slurred speech, and a craving for sweet, starchy foods. "All I want to do in winter," she said, "is go to bed and eat candy."
- Louise, a woman in her mid-fifties. She reported that she noticed signs of depression every year beginning in the fall. Once her mood started to interfere with her ability to work, she would seek medical attention and place herself under the care of a psychiatrist. She believed there must be "something buried in the past" that caused her to hate winter. After several months, however, with the return of spring, she felt that her burden had been lifted and, despite the advice of her therapist, she would terminate therapy. Come fall, however, the depression would return, and once again, her spirit broken, she would return for counseling.

Such a pattern had persisted, she reported, for over a dozen years.

- Margaret, 38 years old. She dreaded the coming of Christmas because "everyone else is running around celebrating and partying and I just want to crawl into a cave and stay there." Margaret was nicknamed "Little Mary Sunshine" by her husband because she would go around turning on every light in the house. He would follow her and turn them off again, unsuspecting that she was inadvertently doing one of the best things possible to improve her condition.
- Nat, 29 years old. During college he had studied to fulfill his dream of becoming a teacher. As he put it, he wanted "to show kids how amazing the world really is." As a SAD patient, however, he found himself virtually incapacitated during the winter months—lethargic, cranky, and irritable, hardly desirable qualities in his chosen profession. Dismayed, he took an entirely different track in his career and became a night-shift data entry supervisor for a polling firm. He remarked, "I can stay in the corner and be left alone, and the computer doesn't care what mood I'm in." He hated his work, he said, but changing jobs had been one of the adaptations he had been forced to make to cope with his condition.
- Naomi, 32 years old. During the winter she was overwhelmed with a desire to sleep—"I just want to hibernate," she moaned. Because we have found that limiting the amount of sleep actually helps SAD patients, we advised her husband to put a lock on the bedroom door to keep her from sleeping during the day.

Basically, our approach to diagnosing SAD is no different than the steps taken to identify any other mental disorder. We obtain a detailed history in order to learn when the symptoms first appeared and how they have affected the person's life. We examine the patient carefully to rule out the presence of physical illness, since a number of diseases produce symptoms that mimic depression. Then we administer standard psychiatric tests designed to quantify the nature of the illness. Depending on our findings, we then initiate treatment with medications, psychotherapy, phototherapy, or some combination of these strategies.

Throughout the process, particularly during the history-taking, we stay especially alert in order to pick up small but significant clues about the seasonal pattern of depression. Oftentimes the patient is not even aware of the yearly cycle. Sometimes a family member or friend supplies us with an observation about the patient that alerts us to the possible presence of SAD. Sometimes we discover clues only after observing the patient over the course of weeks or even months.

One feature often stands out, however, as a sign that we may be dealing with SAD. In these cases, the patient may have been treated by many different psychiatrists and with many different medications, yet has demonstrated only a partial response to therapy. Depending on other factors, it is sometimes possible to make a diagnosis of SAD based almost entirely on the patient's previous response—or rather the lack of response—to medication. The process of diagnosing and treating SAD will be discussed later in greater detail.

Because of the efforts made over the past few years by many talented, dedicated physicians and scientists at institutions in this country and abroad, we now have a very clear picture of what Seasonal Affective Disorder is and how it can be managed. The purpose of this book is to present a definition of SAD, describe its symptoms and their impact on SAD patients, explain the biological dysfunctions that cause the condition, demonstrate how SAD is diagnosed, and outline the course of therapy.

We should note, however, that the process of understanding this condition is an ongoing one. Even as this is being written, research is under way to help refine our knowledge about SAD and to improve our understanding of its treatment. Within the next few years, we should learn a great deal more about how our environment—temperature, climate, humidity, light, air quality—shapes our psyches, and how, by being aware of the natural daily and annual rhythms of our bodies, we can improve our sense of mental and physical well-being.

In the next chapter we will take a closer look at the symptoms of SAD and how the disorder disrupts the lives of those who suffer from it.

CHAPTER 2

THE SYMPTOMS OF SAD

In the early 1980s, a handful of innovative psychiatric researchers identified a new form of mood disorder, one that was triggered by the change of seasons and that possessed a pattern of symptoms clearly distinguishable from other forms of depression. Within a short time they defined the disorder, initiated research into its biological origins, studied scores of patients afflicted with the illness, and developed an innovative approach to therapy that offered hope for those with the illness. After some wrangling and fine-tuning, the researchers settled on a name: Seasonal Affective Disorder.

So thorough and convincing was their work that only six years later, in 1987, SAD was recognized as a true mental disorder by the American Psychiatric Association. SAD is now listed in the *Diagnostic and Statistical Manual of Mental Disorders,* Third Edition, Revised, the psychiatric handbook known as the DSM-III-R. By way of contrast, it should be noted that since the first edition of the DSM appeared in 1952, a considerable number of other mental disorders have been defined by capable researchers, yet many of these have failed to be accepted by the profession. We mention this to give some indication of the close scrutiny given to identification of a mental disorder before it is included in the official nomenclature of psychiatry.

The swiftness with which SAD achieved this official level of recognition underscores the unambiguous validity of the illness: SAD does exist; it possesses a distinctive pattern of symptoms that can be clearly and objectively recognized; it causes suffering in a large number of people; and *it can be treated*.

Over the past few years, researchers and clinicians here and abroad have studied hundreds of SAD patients. To be sure, there are differences in some of the details that have emerged from such studies. As we mentioned, we see and treat most of our patients suffering from more severe symptoms on an inpatient basis, and thus virtually always incorporate antidepressant medication into our treatment plan. In contrast, physicians who treat mostly outpatients have reported good results using just light therapy alone. In some cases, the way in which patients were recruited for treatment—whether through articles placed in local media or through referrals from other physicians, as happens in our practice—has affected the overall statistical picture. In our case, for example, the patients studied tended to be those who had been treated previously and for long periods of time.

However, taken as a whole, the body of available information provides a remarkably consistent picture of the population with SAD. Thus, while much of the information we are about to present was generated through our dealings with patients at Fair Oaks, it is fair to say that similar conclusions can be drawn about SAD patients in other parts of the world, ranging from Norway to New Zealand to Nome, Alaska.

There is no doubt that SAD afflicts many more women than men. The ratio is at least three to one with some researchers reporting that SAD occurs up to five times as often in women.

The disorder can strike at any age. Typically, however, the age of onset ranges from 15 to 30; the average age is 23. It can also occur in children, but is harder to detect, as we'll see shortly. In recounting the history of their illness, almost all patients tell a similar story: Around age 20 (although the event may occur anywhere between puberty and age 27), they became aware that they disliked, felt anxious about, or even dreaded the coming of winter. According to one study, 9 percent of adult patients reported noticing that their SAD symptoms began before age 11; a third of those questioned noted that the problem began before age 19. In contrast, some other types of depression that recur in cycles but are not connected to the change of seasons tend to begin later in life. Some experts feel that the younger age of onset may be a clue that can help distinguish SAD from other forms of depression, but at Fair Oaks we have not necessarily found this to be true.

Roughly five years after the problem starts, it dawns on the patient that symptom patterns have actually persisted for some time. In some cases patients don't seek treatment of SAD until they reach the age of 40, after the syndrome has become progressively worse and more disruptive. The average age of our patients at the time of their first SAD evaluation is 35. However, we should state again that, because our practice is hospital-based, most of our SAD patients have been treated for depression, especially with medication, for many years before the existence of their seasonal disorder is recognized.

The symptoms of SAD can start anytime between September and January. About 30 percent of the patients reported that their depression began in November, while another 30 percent noticed that it began in December. Although remission can begin at any point between January and May, more than half of the patients experienced remission of symptoms in March, and by April, 75 percent have improved.

Reports indicate that anywhere from 10 to 100 percent of SAD patients in any given study had been hospitalized previously for depression. The use of antidepressant medications also falls within a broad range. Most of our patients have received such medications; other studies indicate that, on average, 24 percent of SAD patients had been given antidepressants, 17 percent lithium, and 21 percent thyroid treatments prior to therapy with light.

A family history of affective disorders such as depression was reported by nearly seven out of ten patients. Perhaps one out of four or five recalled that a parent, or perhaps an aunt or uncle, also experienced symptoms similar to SAD. Such evidence strongly supports the notion that SAD springs from some kind of genetic malfunction that is passed from one generation to another. More research is needed, however, to determine the biological basis for the disorder.

Statistically speaking, approximately one in five Americans experiences some form of severe clinical mood disorder at some point in life. At any given moment, perhaps one person in twenty is suffering from depression. Seasonal mood changes, however, form a somewhat different pattern. Overall, perhaps 70 percent of the population experiences some degree of fluctuation in mood and energy level that can be attributed to the shifting seasons. About 20 percent think of these changes as being somewhat problematic; these are people who are perhaps likely to describe themselves as suffering from "winter blues."

In contrast, genuine SAD is believed to occur on a much smaller scale. Estimates of the number of true SAD patients ranges from less than 1 to 2 percent of the population. While this percentage may sound small, it translates into the fact that two and a half to five million Americans find themselves significantly impaired for a significant portion of each year.

As mentioned, women with SAD outnumber men by at least three to one. Frequently these women also experience severe cyclic mood changes that occur at the same time as their menstrual periods. In fact, as a rule, women with past or current psychiatric illness—principally affective disorders, such as depression or anxiety—experience the discomforts of menstruation more severely than normal individuals.

SAD has many features in common with Pre-Menstrual Syndrome (PMS), more technically known as Late Luteal Phase Dysphoric Disorder. Symptoms common to both include the tendency to overeat, craving for carbohydrates, fatigue, lethargy, and sleep disturbance, including excessive sleepiness, technically known as hypersomnia. Often a patient believes that PMS is her only problem, when in fact she has been experiencing depressive symptoms of varying intensity throughout her entire cycle. With SAD—and, for that matter, with other types of depression—the symptoms may grow more severe premenstrually, thus causing confusion as to the real nature of the problem. The medical literature contains many reports of known sufferers of PMS whose doctors failed to detect their depression (seasonal or otherwise) because the symptoms manifested themselves at the same time as their periods. Only after these patients have been treated, however, did they come to realize the extent to which symptoms of depression had been present all along.

The main way that physicians differentiate between SAD and menstrually related syndromes is by analyzing the pattern of symptoms. For example, the condition known as dysmenorrhea, or painful menses, causes pain and discomfort that persist only during the time of actual menstrual discharge, whereas PMS produces a number of additional symptoms that begin premenstrually and remit a few days after the onset of menses. The symptoms of SAD, however, continue to persist for weeks and months on end.

The connection between SAD and a woman's reproductive cycle can be seen in other revealing statistics. Studies of SAD-afflicted women have shown that the birthdates of their children reach a peak in May and decline between August and December. This contrasts sharply with the pattern of the normal population, in which births reach a peak in September and display much less seasonal variation. Such a finding implies that fewer babies are conceived during the months of December and March—the very time during which SAD patients experience decreased energy, diminished sexual drive, and depression.

Many women experience a period of depression following the birth of a child; post-partum depression, as it is known, is the product of many emotional and physical factors, not least of which is the combined effects of the intense hormonal changes the body undergoes during pregnancy and after birth. Many of the women we have treated for SAD report a history in which their seasonal depression began, or perhaps worsened to the point where it was finally recognized, only after the birth of a child, and not necessarily the first child.

Apart from age and sex, what other factors contribute to the existence of SAD? Is there, for example, a "SAD personality"—a type of person prone to develop this disorder? Actually, some evidence seems to suggest that there may be. For example, SAD patients are more likely to describe themselves as "evening types" than a control population. Dr. Al Lewy of the National Institute of Mental Health describes these people appropriately, if somewhat whimsically, as "owls"; their counterparts, the morning people, are likewise known as "larks." Owls are people who find it difficult to function in the morning, who don't really hit their stride until late afternoon or evening. Larks, by contrast, rise singing with the sun and usually turn in early. Owl behavior, like SAD, may arise from the fact that one's internal biological rhythms are operating on different cycles. For owls, biological "morning" may not arrive until two in the afternoon; bedtime, therefore, is shifted to the wee hours. Such lack of harmony between body time and clock time seems to produce many of the symptoms associated with affective disorders.

One thing we've noticed about our SAD patients is the striking change in their personalities between summer and winter. As a rule, we have found that SAD patients are fun people to know and be with—during the sunny months, that is. Then they are lively, creative, sociable beings. Consequently the depression they suffer in winter is even more overwhelming by virtue of its contrast to their summertime mood. Interestingly, too, SAD patients are generally hard-working, productive people. The impact of the disorder is experienced less as melancholy than as an extreme drop in their ability to concentrate or think creatively. One common complaint made by SAD patients is that they don't feel nearly as alert or sharp as they do at other times of the year—a subjective experience that physicians can confirm objectively just by meeting and talking to these patients over the course of time.

Another trait we have noticed is that SAD patients tend to be people who respond to the level of stimulation present in their environment. Thus, if they can somehow force themselves to become socially active during depressed times, they will usually "perk up" and start to feel better. Such social interaction becomes therapeutic in itself, resulting in improved mood. It does not, however, alleviate the long-term effects of the syndrome.

SAD AND CHILDREN

As noted earlier, SAD can occur at an early age. However, many of its symptoms—mood changes, changes in appetite and weight—are easily confused with the physical and emotional turmoil that is a normal part of growing up. Consequently the existence of SAD in a child or adolescent is easily overlooked.

To some extent, the experience of SAD can be the same for both children and adults. Both groups report such signs as fatigue, irritability, carbohydrate cravings, and difficulty rising in the morning. Many find it difficult to move quickly during the day, a symptom known technically as psychomotor retardation. There are some telltale differences, however. For example, while sadness has occasionally been reported as a symptom by children with this disorder, it is not usually the *major* complaint, as it is in many adult patients. Instead, SAD may manifest itself in the form of increased difficulty in getting along with teachers and classmates. In some cases, crying spells have been reported.

According to a recent study of patients under the age of 18, SAD was experienced as sadness, anxiety, or irritability lasting at least two weeks and accompanied by three or more of these symptoms: fatigue, changes in sleep patterns, increased or decreased appetite, craving for carbohydrates, and headaches. Each of the children studied experienced some decrease in the ability to function, measured in terms of difficulties at school or a withdrawal from normal social contacts. One other common thread was found: The symptoms remitted with the arrival of spring or summer. As you might guess, such seasonal changes in attitude might lead an observer to conclude, wrongly, that the child suffered not from a seasonal mood disorder but from a dislike of school.

Another survey, conducted among 1,000 students at a high school in Minnesota, revealed that 6.5 percent of these pupils suffered from SAD. The most frequently noticed symptom was irritability: The kids picked fights and didn't know why.

As Dr. Norman Rosenthal, one of the country's foremost SAD researchers, has observed, SAD can be particularly cruel for a young person. Adults are usually more able to recognize the fact—either from their own perceptions or after having been shown by others—that their mood swings are the result of some kind of internal upheaval. Children and adolescents, in contrast, perceive mood swings as changes that are taking place in the external world. A SAD child might breeze through a certain homework assignment in September, whereas in December, with irritability high and energy low, the child confronted with the same task might protest that the teacher is being "unfair." Similarly, parental demands that the child complete certain chores might be met with surprising resistance. "My parents expect too much of me" is a common lament of young SAD patients. The tipoff that a child is suffering from SAD and not from normal adolescent anxiety is the distinct seasonal pattern of the symptoms involved.

We should note, too, that SAD is not the same as a child's natural tendency to dislike school. One way to distinguish SAD from "school phobia" is that dislike of school is usually noted early on as the fall term begins, whereas the onset of SAD occurs somewhat later, as winter approaches.

As we will see in later chapters, an important component in the treatment of SAD in adolescents is the same as for adults: bright, full-spectrum lights administered under a regimen prescribed by a physician. The response to phototherapy in young people can in fact be particularly dramatic. In terms of grades, for example, many SAD-afflicted students who in academic terms could barely keep their heads above water—above C level, so to speak—find that after light therapy their enthusiasm and ability to concentrate return. Many go on to make the honor rolls at their schools. After a course of light therapy, one young athlete found that his physical sluggishness had disappeared, as evidenced by an improvement in his swimming times.

THE GEOGRAPHY OF SAD

Of course, the further north you go, the higher the incidence of SAD is likely to be. A study conducted by one researcher, for example, has found that perhaps 25 percent of the population in northerly latitudes is affected by at least some of the SAD symptoms, especially weight gain and excessive daytime fatigue. Also, further north, SAD symptoms appear earlier and remit later in the year than they do in more southern climes.

SAD patients report the influence of latitude on their symptoms in a number of unexpected ways. Many times patients have told us that they returned, all smiles, from their winter vacations in Florida or Jamaica, only to be plunged into depression a few days later. Another physician described a patient who said that while living in Morocco and Egypt, her depressions began a month later and were less severe than while living in the northeastern United States. This person had also lived in Chile, and had noticed that her "down times" began in June and ended in September, the months corresponding to winter south of the equator.

Some SAD patients have refused to travel to northern cities during the winter, even when required to do so by their employers, because they knew they would be unable to function if they subjected themselves to a colder, darker climate, even for just a few days.

If we may coin a phrase, in patients with SAD, latitude is attitude. As one noted researcher, Dr. Thomas Wehr, stated, it seems as if there is a "biological equator" that helps define our point of mental and physical equilibrium. For people who are hypersensitive to seasonal changes in light, travel in one direction or the other can disrupt the fragile balance of their circadian cycles.

The impact of northern winters on humans may be a vestige

of our evolutionary history. After all, our species probably began in a lush, sunny climate—Syria, perhaps, or Africa. As we spread across the globe, our early evolution took place in such Mediterranean regions as the Middle East, Egypt, or southern France. Migrating into the colder, darker regions of northern Europe must have taken more of an evolutionary toll on our forebears; SAD may be part of a genetic legacy that renders some people less tolerant of a harsher climate than those who stayed closer to their lands of origin.

A survey conducted by the newspaper *USA Today* revealed, not very surprisingly, that states with higher northern latitude, a higher number of cloudy days, and generally lower temperatures reported the highest incidence of SAD. Latitude was found to be by far the most important of these elements in determining the severity of the disorder. In fact, some studies show that Northerners are ten times more likely than others to develop a case of SAD. Furthermore, the farther north you go, the sooner winter depression sets in. In our own region of the country, most people with SAD reported that their symptoms usually began in late October or November and began to remit in February or March. As you go south, however, depressive episodes begin later and remit earlier.

Natives and residents of Alaska are accustomed to the experience of seasonal changes in mood and energy. At the other extreme, Dr. Daniel F. Kripke of the University of California at San Diego reports being frustrated in his attempts to study the disorder because there is a severe lack of SAD patients in that sunny part of the country! San Diego experiences 300 sunny days a year; by contrast, parts of New England are lucky if they have 65 days of sunshine in twelve months.

The increased incidence of SAD with increased latitude is a phenomenon that has been noted elsewhere in the world as well. A magazine survey conducted in Norway asked readers to respond to fifteen questions about winter moods. If they had eight or more positive answers (for example, "Yes, I feel tired in winter") they were asked to send in their surveys for analysis. Significantly more surveys were returned from the three northernmost counties in Norway—situated partly or completely above the Arctic circle—than from the southern regions. And studies of Norwegians reveal a high incidence of sleep disturbances, as well as abnormal physiological symptoms such as increased secretion of cortisol and growth hormone, which are believed to be symptoms of stress related to wintertime light deprivation.

At the other end of the world, a physician preparing to spend a year with a small group of researchers in Antarctica, boned up on many different medical skills, ranging from dentistry to surgery. He was particularly aware that he would be called on primarily to handle complaints of depression, especially during the six months of winter darkness.

Recently medical professionals in New Zealand have begun to study the incidence of SAD in their country. It is interesting to note that New Zealand is about as far south of the equator as Rockville, Maryland, home of the National Institute of Mental Health (NIMH), is north of it. The results of a survey of patients with SAD, when compared with results from NIMH studies, found strikingly similar patterns in virtually every aspect: age and sex of patients, severity of symptoms, climatic conditions.

Before we move on to a discussion of symptoms, let us make some further comments about the importance of geography in SAD. Much of the effect that latitude has on the incidence and severity of SAD is related to the way sunlight strikes the earth. This in turn is governed by three basic facts about our planet: its generally spherical shape, the fact that it is tilted on its axis, and the fact that it travels around the sun over the course of a year. As you may remember from high school science, light from the sun strikes the equator essentially head on. As you travel north or south, the curvature of the earth causes sunlight to strike at a more glancing angle; thus the amount of sunlight that would cover a square foot in, say, a South American country like Ecuador, is "stretched out" to cover a much greater area in, say, Madison, Wisconsin. Consequently those regions must make do with less sunlight and less heat.

Similarly, sunlight must penetrate the earth's atmosphere

before it strikes the ground. The gases and dust that make up the air diffuse a great deal of the energy from sunlight. At the equator, the atmosphere (more precisely that portion of it comprised of the troposphere and the stratosphere, including the ozone layer) is less than thirty miles deep. However, to penetrate to, say, Washington D.C., sunlight strikes at more of an angle, and must therefore travel a greater distance—closer to sixty miles—before reaching the ground. As a result, the atmosphere diffuses a higher degree of radiant energy, leaving less sunlight to penetrate to the surface.

One final note: Despite popular belief to the contrary, the earth is actually closer to the sun during our northern winter than during our summer. The coldness of winter is not the result of distance from the sun; instead, it is caused by the fact that the northern hemisphere tilts backward, away from the sun, during those months. In fact, in the northern third of the United States, the total amount of ultraviolet (warming) radiation that reaches the ground in December is only about one-fifteenth of the amount present in June.

This severe wintertime drop in available ultraviolet radiation may turn out to be an extremely significant factor in the onset—and treatment—of SAD, a topic we will return to in Chapter 6.

THE SYMPTOMS OF SAD

In the preceding pages we have mentioned briefly the symptoms that define SAD as a recognizable illness. Let's look at those symptoms more closely now, to see how they affect the lives of those who experience them.

Between 1981 and 1985, the National Institute of Mental Health surveyed over 150 patients with SAD and developed a statistical profile of the disorder. Among the findings:

- An overwhelming 96 percent of SAD patients reported decreased activity in the winter.

- A similar number (94 percent) stated that interpersonal problems—relationships with spouses, lovers, family members, friends, and coworkers—occurred during these months.
- Of the vast majority who reported changes in mood, most (96 percent) noted feelings of sadness accompanied by anxiety (84 percent) and irritability (79 percent).
- Difficulties at work were mentioned by 88 percent of the patients.
- Only one patient detected no change in appetite. In contrast, two out of three patients experienced an increase, while another 19 percent noticed a decrease. Another group of patients—14 percent—noticed that their appetites fluctuated: elevated on some days and diminished on others. For women, this fluctuation may occur premenstrually, thus further confusing the border between PMS and SAD. In a subgroup of 123 patients, some 67 percent reported an increased craving for carbohydrates.
- As a consequence of these altered eating patterns, most patients noted a change in their overall body weight. More than seven out of ten, for example, noticed an increase, while another 13 percent lost weight. One percent of those studied found their weight rose and fell over time. However, 15 percent reported no change in weight.
- More than six out of ten patients reported that their sexual drive had dropped. Furthermore, 61 percent of 116 women noted added difficulties with their menstrual cycles, including increased severity of PMS symptoms.
- It is surprising to note that, out of a subgroup of 71 patients, 53 of them found that their symptoms of depression improved dramatically as they traveled closer to the equator.
- As a rule, the symptoms of SAD occurred gradually over a period of weeks, rather than striking all at once.

As you can tell from these numbers, most SAD patients experience many different symptoms as part of their condition. Because several of these symptoms occur simultaneously in the same patient, they are said to constitute a syndrome that should alert physicians to the presence of the disorder. In this regard, SAD is like other serious psychiatric illnesses, most of which are identified by a pattern of many different symptoms.

Our point in mentioning this is to stress the fact that, as a rule, treating the individual symptom will not result in improvement of the condition. To illustrate: You might take an antihistamine to relieve your runny nose, but such medication does nothing to eliminate the underlying cause of your cold. By analogy, using psychiatric counseling for SAD might help a patient cope with difficulties encountered in maintaining personal relationships but would overlook the fact that such difficulties stemmed from mood swings attributable to the lack of exposure to bright light. As we proceed, then, keep in mind that each individual symptom of SAD forms just part of the whole picture.

Mood Changes

One of our patients, a 45-year-old woman named Olivia, told us that every fall, with the turning of the leaves, she senses a creeping form of terror. She starts to feel "anxious about everything in general and nothing in particular"; by winter she is "absolutely miserable." As she puts it, "I turn into a holy terror—cranky, irritable, snapping at everyone. I don't enjoy being with people or going out. All I want to do is sleep the day away.

"Most of the time I feel so sad, and for no reason at all that I can make out. Nothing seems to cheer me up. I could watch the funniest movie ever made and not even crack a smile. I can barely function at work, and that makes me feel edgy, because it seems like any minute I could lose my job. That just makes me feel worse. I'm glad my husband has the patience of a saint, because it seems like every year I tell him my New Year's resolution is to divorce him. He doesn't react. He knows that come April or May I'll be my old lovable self again."

Olivia is a typical SAD patient. Her winter depressions are characterized by sadness and irritability. Her mood changes make her almost intolerable to herself as well as to those around her. By summer, however, she becomes more energetic and socially outgoing. Her mood becomes as sunny as a cloudless day in June.

The connection between seasons and mood has been noted since ancient times. The Greek physician Hippocrates, who lived around 400 B.C., observed, "If any violent change occurred in the air according to the seasons, the brain also becomes different from what it was."

Many of these seasonal mood changes are no more serious than a case of transient cabin fever, the result of being cooped up and inactive because of the vicissitudes of winter weather or the stresses of year-end holidays. For patients with SAD, however, mood fluctuations are directly attributable to the reduction in environmental light. Even in summertime, a deterioration in mood can occur if a patient moves to an office without windows, or if there is an extended period of cloudy weather.

One problem we face in managing SAD is that seasonally related mood changes are perceived, by patients and nonpatients alike, to be "understandable." That is, they are the "natural" result of one's particular circumstances. For example, during the fall, when children return to school, a mother may begin to feel an added level of stress as she copes with the pressure of a new morning routine. Then, with the onset of the holiday season, she may begin to feel an increased level of sadness. With the arrival of the warmer days of spring, her improved mood is chalked up to her "hope" for the summer. As we have seen, however, attributing these mood changes to external events overlooks the true underlying, internal cause of the symptoms and can lead to delays in diagnosing and treating the condition.

One study found that 19 out of 23 SAD patients experienced a change in mood within a few days after traveling to sunnier regions of the world, including Florida and the Caribbean. For some patients, the change occurred as soon as they walked off the plane. Predictably, their moods worsened upon returning north.

For most SAD patients, mood changes are, at the very least, annoying and disruptive. For a small number, however, the feeling of sadness can become quite troubling. In some patients, thoughts of suicide occur; these thoughts may even lead to actual suicide attempts.

Olivia also mentioned anxiety, a symptom we have found to be one of the most prominent features of this disorder. At this point we should make it clear that there are two types of anxiety associated with SAD. One type, as illustrated by Olivia and Jenny, whom we met in Chapter 1, is known as anticipatory anxiety, so called because it describes the fear, or the anticipation, that something is about to go wrong. When the seasons begin to change, many SAD patients become anxious not because of any immediately recognizable cause but because they know that at some point in the near future they will start to feel bad. In a sense, anticipatory anxiety is a form of learned behavior that becomes entrenched as the SAD cycle repeats itself over the course of years.

The other type of anxiety is directly related to the depression itself. In other words, once the symptoms of SAD have appeared, patients may then begin to feel anxious about the ways in which the disorder is beginning to upset their lives, their families, and their ability to work. At this point the depression and the anxiety are intricately connected. This form of anxiety no longer represents an anticipatory reaction, but reflects a component of the mood change that is rooted within the biological disruptions caused by SAD.

In the next chapter we'll discuss more thoroughly the role of light in regulating the secretions of body chemicals that control our moods. At this point, though, we should mention something that we will stress repeatedly throughout the book: Like any medical therapy, use of light to treat mood problems is not a do-it-yourself affair; it should be handled only by a qualified psychiatrist or other medical professional.

Changes in Appetite

For Paula, a 42-year-old publicity agent for a computer manufacturer, the approach of winter means she is about to enter what she calls her "squirrel phase." As she describes it, "I go into stores and buy box after box of holiday cookies and loaf after loaf of bread. I stash everything away in the freezer, on the shelves, anywhere there's room. I'm like a squirrel storing up nuts. I pretend I do it because I'm getting ready for Christmas visits from friends and relatives, but that's not true. I do it to have stuff on hand to satisfy my cravings. It's all I can do to keep myself from scarfing down every last crumb."

Another SAD patient, a 29-year-old journalist named Robert, remarked that "in the winter I turn Italian." He eats heaping platefuls of spaghetti at virtually every meal. He describes his craving as "uncontrollable." Interestingly, though, he says that in the summer he "can barely stand to look a plate of pasta in the face."

Paula and Robert illustrate one of the predominant features of SAD: a seasonal change in eating habits, usually seen as an increase in appetite that prompts a craving for carbohydrates. Typically, of course, most people experience a change of menu during the colder months—eating more hot dishes, such as noodles or chili, or eating fewer salads and fruits because of the limited availability of fresh produce. But for SAD patients, the dietary changes are extreme. Such people mention specifically an increased intake of pasta, breads, pastries, potatoes, chips, chocolates, and candy during the winter months. Their intake of caffeinated beverages also rises substantially. Generally speaking, some SAD patients seem to crave starches, while others prefer sugary items. Obviously, such a diet can affect body weight, which in turn can cause a decrease in self-esteem, a cycle of symptoms we'll cover shortly.

While most SAD patients notice an increase in appetite, a few notice that their desire for food actually wanes in the winter. Only a small minority detect no fluctuation in eating habits at all.

Most SAD patients do not describe the increased intake of

food as a pleasurable experience. On the contrary, in discussing the problem they use the word "compulsion," or mention the "pressure to eat." When asked why they eat so much, many will say they do so "to get more energy," or "to keep warm," or "to perk myself up." One woman told us glumly that she feels so depressed in the winter that she'll do anything she can to make herself happy. As she put it, "I don't care about my diet, I don't care how I look. If eating a quart of ice cream and a bag of chocolate chip cookies will make me feel better, then by God I'm going to eat it."

As with other SAD symptoms, appetite returns to normal in spring and summer. Typically, SAD patients who gorged themselves on bread and potatoes in December are eating less food—usually a diet of fruits, vegetables, and salads—by June.

As physicians, it is our responsibility to assess the nature of these changes in eating habits in order to rule out the possibility that the patient is suffering from some form of eating disorder, rather than from SAD or some other mental or physical illness. An increased desire for carbohydrates, for example, is often associated with premenstrual syndrome, as well as such disorders as hypothyroidism and hypoglycemia. Screening patients for these other conditions is a routine part of the general psychiatric evaluation.

Why should people with SAD experience these cravings for carbohydrates? What inner mechanism compels them to consume vast quantities of high-calorie foods? Surprisingly, such behavior may actually be the result of the body's attempts to improve its own mood. Carbohydrate-rich foods appear to accelerate the production of serotonin, a brain chemical—technically known as a neurotransmitter—that carries signals across the gaps between brain cells. Serotonin is believed to play an important role in alleviating depression. Thus, by increasing their intake of carbohydrates, SAD patients may actually be following the body's orders to provide the raw materials needed to increase the supply of serotonin and thus improve mood, a process we'll describe in more detail in the next chapter. In addition to its other effects, light therapy helps to restore balance to the patient's appetite by bringing carbohydrate cravings under control. In one study, patients reported that after ten days of phototherapy their appetites—their general desire for food—had diminished only slightly, but their cravings for sweet, starchy foods had fallen by 50 percent.

One other point worth mentioning: Researchers have found that changes in diet have an effect on sleep patterns, and not just on total length of sleep, but the amount of time spent in deep sleep or in the dream phase as well. They conclude that some of the sleep changes noticed in SAD patients may be the result not of SAD itself, but of the dietary impact the disorder can have. A discussion of sleep symptoms appears later in this chapter.

Changes in Body Weight

We first saw Tracy in January 1987, when she came to Fair Oaks seeking help for depression. We were somewhat surprised when she told us she was an aerobics instructor; she seemed out of shape and overweight. She told us that she had, in fact, gained over twenty pounds since November.

Tracy burst into tears as she told her story. Two years earlier, in the spring of 1985, she had moved from her native Florida to New Jersey when her husband, Vince, was transferred to another job. A friendly, vivacious person, Tracy quickly made new friends and began teaching exercise classes at a fitness club. When fall arrived, however, she began to feel moody and depressed. She remembered "gorging" herself on doughnuts and cupcakes—"junk I never used to touch." Her weight shot up; she became lethargic and grouchy.

"One day," she said, "I was leading a class and I happened to catch a glance of myself in the mirror. I was horrified by what I saw—I was becoming fat and puffy. I was in no shape to be telling people how to stay fit. I burst into tears and left the class. I told my husband that relocating must have been harder on me than I realized, and that I needed some time to get myself back together. A few days later I packed my bags and returned to my parents' home in Tampa. I stayed there the rest of the winter. By March, though, I felt one hundred percent better. I missed Vince so much that I came back to New Jersey.

"Things were fine for a long time. Then, around Thanksgiving, the same thing happened again. I put on weight. I had to buy a bunch of new clothes. And I cried a lot. Sometimes it seemed like just dragging my fat body out of bed and getting it dressed was a full day's work. I feel this irresistible need to sleep, but on those days when I do sleep more, my symptoms just seem to get worse.

"Now I'm really torn—I want to go back to Florida, but Vince wants to stay here. I don't think my marriage can stand another long separation. And when I think about getting divorced, I get so sad I can hardly stand it."

Tracy's story illustrates one of the physical consequences of Seasonal Affective Disorder that many patients find to be the most troubling: fluctuation in body weight. In her case, gaining twenty pounds or more was particularly disruptive. Normally healthy and physically fit, she felt compelled to give up her career, and possibly her marriage, to escape the consequences of the northern winter—hardly a recommended remedy.

The seasonal pattern of her symptoms, of course, was the clue that led us to suspect, and quickly diagnose, the presence of SAD.

At Fair Oaks, we have noticed that many of our SAD patients report "considerable" winter weight gains—anywhere from five to twenty-five pounds or more, with the typical gain being about ten pounds. One patient consistently put on fifty pounds between September and December! Such increases create a financial burden as well. Patients buy more food of course, but, even more importantly, many patients must buy additional clothes to accommodate their larger bulk. Many report that, like people with eating disorders, they own two sets of clothes: a "fat wardrobe" and a "thin wardrobe."

Obviously, increased weight in SAD patients is a product of increased consumption of high-calorie foods coupled with poor self-image and a decreased level of energy and activity. It is possible that the body is triggering these changes in appetite and weight as a form of self-protection. Adding weight in the winter, for example, may be another holdover from our evolutionary past: Increased bulk helped our cave-dwelling ancestors to cope with cold winter weather. In modern times, with heated homes replacing damp caves, such protectionary measures are at best unnecessary and, as in Tracy's case, counterproductive.

Weight changes complicate the SAD picture in another way. Understandably, SAD patients, like most people, can be sensitive about physical appearance. When their weight goes up, their self-esteem goes down. They don't want anyone to look at them; they don't want to appear in public; they may grow to hate themselves. Such feelings contribute to their desire to withdraw from activities with family and friends. Social withdrawal contributes to their feelings of depression, which may trigger another carbohydrate-eating binge, causing more weight gain, and so on in a vicious circle.

In many cases patients are able to diet in the spring and lose the weight they gained over the winter. As the years pass, however, many find it harder and harder to lose the added pounds. For some people the weight gained because of SAD becomes a permanent and unwelcome fixture, thus damaging their sense of self-esteem even further.

Changes in Energy Level and Sleep Patterns

At Fair Oaks a majority of our SAD patients tell us that they sleep considerably more in the winter than they do in the summer. Typically, people who normally sleep for eight hours might find themselves sleeping ten, twelve, even fourteen hours a night. The tragedy is that, even with this additional sleep, the patient still awakens feeling tired and unrested.

Several of our patients have told us they are so concerned about falling asleep at the wheel of a car that they can't even drive during the winter. One patient, a 33-year-old woman named Yvonne, said she dreaded attending the daily conferences required in her job as program director for a classical music radio station. "I can't stay interested, I can't concentrate.

I just want to fall asleep," she told us. As one fatigued patient put it, "I drag myself through my day at work, hating my job, myself, and everyone around me. I get home, gorge myself on pasta, and sleep for twelve hours. The next morning I wake up feeling tired and horrible and force myself to get through another day."

A similar story was told by a college student, a 20-year-old named Amy. In winter her pattern was to sleep anywhere from 12 to 16 hours a day. At the height of the season—perhaps we should say the depth—Amy would miss between two and three weeks of classes because, she said, "I simply couldn't drag myself out of bed." During this time, she said, "I just turn into a bowl of mush. I feel weak. I can't function. I have no motivation or energy. I know my brain's there, but you wouldn't know it, because I can't think clearly. My thoughts come slowly and I can't concentrate on anything."

Interestingly the best way to help alleviate the sleepiness associated with SAD is not to get more sleep but less. As we'll see in the discussion of the treatment of SAD later in the book, limiting sleep to eight or nine hours a night and cutting out naps during the day actually improves the patient's energy level and ability to concentrate. It's often hard to convince patients of this fact, since many of them would rather sleep another three or four hours than be awake and suffer the symptoms of their illness for that much time.

To many people, doctors and patients alike, the symptoms of SAD—excessive eating, weight gain, oversleeping, social withdrawal—resemble the seasonal rhythms of hibernation. Indeed, patients often make remarks that are variations on the theme of "I should have been born a bear," and "During the winter I hibernate." In fact, the striking similarities between SAD and winter dormancy in animals seem to suggest that both conditions are the body's way of conserving energy during the time of year when food is scarce and it takes more effort just to stay warm and active. Also, the body temperature of a hibernating bear will drop dramatically; a human's body temperature may also drop to some extent during the winter. One difference, however, is that animals sleep more deeply during this period. The same cannot be said for SAD patients, as we'll explain later.

SAD affects sleep in a number of specific ways. Using data from electroencephalograph (EEG) tracings, one study of nine SAD patients found that, compared to summer sleep patterns, overall time spent sleeping increased during the winter by an average of 17 percent. It took 23 percent longer for these patients to fall asleep, and there was a surprisingly large drop of nearly 50 percent in the amount of time spent in deep sleep, which is known to be the most restful and restorative phase. These patients also tended to waken more often during the night; if such wakenings last for more than a few moments, the sleeper can become conscious, which lessens the quality of sleep.

Changes in sleep patterns trigger a number of other problems as well. For one thing, when patients sleep longer but awaken unrested, they feel physically and mentally exhausted during every waking hour, but particularly in the morning. Many are concerned that they are suffering from a physical illness, since many SAD symptoms—muscular aches and sensitivity to cold, for example—resemble those of viral illness. Such patients naturally tend to worry when their physicians are unable to identify the cause of the problem. The increased weariness makes them cranky and harder to get along with, a situation that only contributes to their sense of isolation from other people.

Of course, many people suffer from a variety of specific sleep disorders totally unrelated to SAD, which can be specifically recognized and treated by a physician. Some people have trouble falling asleep; others fall asleep too easily. Some people awaken dozens, even hundreds of times a night. Others find it so hard to awaken in the morning that they feel "hung over." Still other people suffer from any one of the many medical conditions—from obstructed breathing to arthritis—that can interfere with the ability to achieve a decent night's rest. In many cases, however, poor sleep is simply the result of poor habits: too much coffee, misuse of "sleeping medications," or overstimulation—physical or emotional—in the hours before bedtime.

In assessing a patient with a sleep problem, we always ask about seasonal patterns. As with other SAD symptoms, sleep difficulties triggered by the disorder begin in the winter and remit during the spring and summer. In addition, the presence of hypersomnia (excessive sleepiness) is another clue that helps us distinguish SAD from other forms of depression. Typically, depressed individuals suffer from interrupted sleep that causes them to awaken early in the morning. In SAD, the opposite problem exists. A more detailed discussion of the various types of depression appears in Chapter 3.

Like other SAD symptoms, sleep changes seem to arise from disturbances in an individual's circadian rhythms. In winter, without adequate sunlight to provide our bodies with the clues they need to maintain proper functioning, physiological events such as the secretion of certain hormones, which usually occurs at a certain point in the day, may be shifted to another time. In hypersomnia, the body rhythms that govern sleep appear to be shifted abnormally from late evening to the wee hours of the morning. Thus patients may fall asleep at odd times. They may then wake up, say, in the evening or be wide awake in the evening and want to stay up because they feel so well. Then they finally turn in about three in the morning. When they wake up they must literally drag themselves out of bed to make it to work.

One chemical suspect involved in sleep disturbances is melatonin, a hormone that has been found to induce sleep in experimental animals. In humans, melatonin—indicted but not yet convicted of being the chief culprit in SAD—is secreted primarily during the hours of darkness. Conversely, animals such as rats who are active at night secrete melatonin during the day.

Some studies indicate that during the long winter nights, we humans generate greater amounts of melatonin. In susceptible individuals, this excess melatonin apparently produces excess sleepiness. And when patients with SAD sleep more hours during the day, they are exposed to even less light. Longer exposure to darkness increases the production of melatonin, a situation that only worsens the problem.

Circadian rhythms also affect the various individual stages of sleep as well. Before we explain how, perhaps we should explain what we mean by the "stages of sleep."

You are probably aware that sleep is not one smooth, continuous period of unconsciousness that begins when we drop off and ends when we open our eyes in the morning. Instead the pattern of sleep—as reflected in the tracings of brain waves recorded by the EEG—demonstrates considerable activity throughout the course of the night. This pattern is referred to as the architecture of sleep.

When we close our eyes, we enter what is known as Stage O, the time of transition from wakefulness to sleep during which the brain is still alert but relaxed. After a few minutes we cross into Stage 1 sleep, lasting a few minutes or so, during which the pulse and respiration become more even. Then we enter Stage 2 sleep, lasting about an hour. At this point we are completely unaware of our surroundings. If someone lifted your eyelids, for example, you would not see anything.

Once EEG tracings reveal that our brains are generating a different pattern of waves, called slow waves, it is an indication we have entered sleep stages 3 and 4. These stages are what we mean by "deep sleep." Periods of deep sleep are of differing lengths, depending on the time of night. Early on, deep sleep may last for an hour or more; toward morning, however, you may sleep deeply for only a few minutes. It takes more energy to awaken from deep sleep than from any other stage. Interestingly, if you are deprived of sleep for, say, a few days, the next night you will spend more time in Stage 4 than any other stage in order to make up the "deficit," a fact that underscores the importance of deep sleep in providing rest and restoration.

After a period of deep sleep, you enter what is known as the rapid eye movement or REM phase, named for its distinctive pattern of eye activity. As you probably know, REM sleep is the period during which we dream. A REM phase can last anywhere from five or ten minutes to an hour; the longer periods occur just before we awaken, which is why our morning dreams sometimes seem so detailed and complex. At the end of a REM phase we awaken briefly—usually not enough to regain consciousness—and begin again at Stage 1.

It takes about ninety minutes to go from Stage 1 to the end of REM. A complete trip through all the stages comprises one sleep cycle. Typically a sleeper will undergo four or five cycles in the course of a night. In each cycle the different stages occupy a slightly different percentage of time: more deep sleep and less REM early on, less deep sleep and more REM toward morning.

The architecture of sleep is governed by circadian rhythms. The onset of the REM phase is closely linked to the body's temperature rhythm. Normally, body temperature drops in the early morning and rises again to a peak just before waking. If the circadian rhythms are disturbed, that peak may occur too soon, and the time it takes to enter the REM phase may become abnormally short. The sleep/wake cycle also follows a rhythmic pattern. If these clocks malfunction, then the patient may experience an abnormal pattern of sleep. In depression, some rhythms are shifted so that they occur earlier than is normal; many depressed individuals thus awaken too soon in the morning. In SAD, however, the opposite is the case: Body temperature rhythms are shifted to a later time, causing hypersomnia and feelings of sleepiness that persist through much of the rest of the day.

At Fair Oaks we have found that the benefits of phototherapy are generally seen without regard to the time of day it is administered. An important exception is that phototherapy during the evening or at night may cause overstimulation, which in turn may cause difficulty in falling asleep. However, some SAD researchers are investigating the possibility that the effectiveness of phototherapy may depend on the exact nature of an individual's circadian pattern. Patients whose circadian rhythms are delayed, for example, might benefit especially from light therapy administered early in the morning in an effort to set the biological clock to an earlier time. It's possible that awareness of these rhythms may turn out to be a crucial factor in designing an effective phototherapeutic regimen for a particular individual. Such theories are still controversial; some SAD researchers are not yet certain that circadian disturbances are an important feature of the disorder. More research is needed to answer many of the unanswered questions that remain about this fascinating subject. In the next chapter we'll discuss circadian rhythms in greater detail.

Other Symptoms

The features of SAD that have been discussed so far occur in the vast majority of patients with the disorder. There are other symptoms that appear with less frequency but which nonetheless pose significant difficulties for those who must cope with the illness.

For example, 62 percent of SAD patients seen by the NIMH over a four-year period reported that their sexual drive, technically known as the libido, had decreased. We've already mentioned that during the winter months, patients with SAD tend to conceive children at a significantly lower rate. For one of my patients, a 26-year-old plumber named Chuck, this decrease in sexual appetite had severe consequences.

Chuck had married his high school sweetheart in April 1986. He described their honeymoon as "pretty wild" and indicated that their level of sexual activity had continued at a high level over the ensuing months. By late fall, however, Chuck began to experience a drop in overall energy level. His sleepiness increased; he began going to bed earlier and sleeping later. Not surprisingly, his interest in sex tapered off as well. Understandably, his wife began to feel that Chuck had lost interest in her. During the arguments that took place between them frequently that winter, she indicated her suspicion that he might be seeing another woman, and that this surreptitious relationship was draining him of his former energy. In January, Chuck and his wife sought help from a marital counselor, who happened to know of Fair Oaks' interest in seasonal depression. Chuck was referred to us, and it wasn't long before his SAD was detected. A regimen of phototherapy helped him regain much of his former sexual interest.

Physical symptoms have been reported in some cases of SAD. For example, many patients complain of aching muscles and bemoan the fact that it takes a tremendous effort to stand, walk, or move. "My arms and legs feel like lead weights," is a typical remark. During our visits with patients we have noted that they actually talk more slowly during depressed times. Their posture and walk also change over time. In the summer they stroll in with shoulders back and chins up; in winter, though, they act as if the earth's gravity had suddenly doubled. As one woman told us, "I slouch into the kitchen and reach for a can on the shelf and it seems like my arm is made of concrete. When I lift my arm it's like a slow-motion movie." She added, in tones of utter self-loathing, "I feel like a slug."

Some patients report other physical problems, such as back pain or headaches, and many blame feelings of depression for increased susceptibility to such winter ailments as colds and flu.

THE SOCIAL IMPACT OF SAD

As you no doubt noticed from the stories of SAD patients, the disorder disrupts life in a number of ways. For the individual, SAD means coping with mood swings, changes in appetite and body weight, decreased energy, diminished interest in life, and numerous associated physical complaints. Because their personalities undergo such radical transformations, SAD patients experience difficulties on the social front as well. These problems can occur in all of the most important areas of life that involve interpersonal relationships: family, work, and friends.

Impact on the Family

A physician in Wisconsin reported that during the spring and summer, a patient named Dolores, a 40-year-old woman, was outgoing and active. She delighted in painting watercolors and enjoyed participating in church activities. With the arrival of fall, however, her church attendance dropped off. "I can barely stand to pick up a paint brush," she remarked. "If I do manage to start a painting, I know I'll never finish. At least, not until spring." Dolores mentioned that she had a great-aunt with a similar problem; the aunt was legendary in her family because of her total refusal to participate in any family activities between Thanksgiving and Easter.

Elizabeth, a real estate agent in her late thirties, told us that with the onset of winter, she felt like "divorcing my whole family." The mere sound of her children's voices "grated on my nerves," she stated. During the dark months she abdicated virtually every one of the domestic responsibilities she handled with ease at other times of year. Naturally, her family was forced to find ways of compensating. Her husband, Ted, did what he could to feed and entertain the kids. He took them skating and to the movies as often as possible—anything, he told her, to keep them out of her hair. He found himself constantly reassuring the kids that "Mommy still loves you," even though at times he began to doubt what he was saying. Sometimes Ted even ended up handling some of Elizabeth's real estate duties—showing a house or talking to a lawyer. He always found an explanation to account for his wife's annual absence at his company's Christmas party, but he knew the office rumor mill was grinding. His resentment toward her grew. He began to wonder if he was somehow responsible for his wife's mood, or if through her behavior she was punishing him in some way for something he had said or done.

This last anecdote illustrates some of the ways SAD can affect the families of those who suffer from the disorder. In fact, almost all patients report some degree of disruption in family life because of the illness. Like any form of depression, SAD can cause a complicated tangle of emotions between patients and their relatives. All too often these emotions are sensed but are chronically suppressed, posing the risk that they will erupt in a destructive outburst.

There is anger—unjustified but real—that the patient is sick and that the illness is disrupting everyone's lives. There is frustration caused by the patient's apparent inability to get well and by the repeating patterns of the disorder. This frustration often takes the form of caustic remarks by relatives: "Why don't you do something to pull yourself out of this?" Resentment arises when relatives are deprived of attention from the spouse or parent. Many times relatives feel a sense of guilt, as if they were somehow responsible for causing the patient's condition. Coupled with guilt is the feeling of inadequacy in coping with the problem. "Life is unfair" is a comment we often hear, from patients and their relatives alike.

During a SAD patient's "down times," arguments and squabbles increase; couples are more often impatient and less tolerant of each other's foibles. Relatives feel they must alter or restrict their activities or behavior; they must "walk on eggshells" or act "super carefully" to avoid exacerbating the patient's condition. They resent the fact that symptoms seem to strike "out of the blue," which makes it difficult to plan activities. Having to change plans suddenly only adds to the bitterness. Similarly, the patient's overreactivity and irritability make it difficult for family members to predict how their afflicted relative will react emotionally or behaviorally to a given situation.

Such misunderstandings about the disease and its effect on patients widen emotional and physical rifts between partners. Many patients have told us that during the darkest times they seriously consider leaving their mates; in one case, a woman's seasonal mood swings were cited by her husband as a grounds for divorce.

For children, a parent's disorder can be particularly scary. It is hard for them to grasp why Mommy loves them on some days and not on others. The transformation of a happy, laughing, and energetic person into a gloomy, short-tempered, lethargic one can be puzzling and frightening to anybody, but especially so to children, who need to trust their parents to provide stability and security in their lives. Many children feel ashamed of a sick parent and avoid bringing friends into the house to play. Children who are old enough to assume the responsibility of caring for the depressed parent may resent the burden placed on them, a burden not shared by younger siblings.

Complicating the SAD picture is the fact that the disorder appears to be hereditary to some degree, as evidenced by Dolores's story, and may be genetically related to other forms of affective illness. For example some studies report that one out of three SAD patients has a parent who experienced similar seasonal mood swings. And more than two out of three have close relatives who suffer from some kind of major affective disorder, such as depression or alcoholism. In some cases patients fear they will pass the illness on to unborn children; they also worry if they see symptoms beginning to emerge in children they already have.

The administration of phototherapy works directly to alleviate the patient's feeling of depression. But it also works indirectly by producing a beneficial effect on the patient's relatives: They perceive that the spouse or parent has "returned" to the family. As we will see in Chapter 7, however, the use of lights is not always sufficient by itself. In Elizabeth's case, for example, months of family therapy were needed to help reknit the tattered fabric of her relationships with her husband and children.

Impact on Work and Careers

One magazine article described a SAD patient who convinced her employer to allow her to work out of her home. During the spring and summer she cranked out work at a feverish pitch, accumulating a stockpile of completed assignments that she would then deliver at regular intervals throughout the rest of the year. Thus the work she handed over in January may actually have been completed the previous July. She was able to create the impression that she was a reliable, productive, year-round worker. The stress of maintaining this facade—long, strenuous hours of work in the summer, followed by isolation and idleness in winter—soon became more than she could handle.

Many patients report that moving from a well-lit to a poorly lit environment can result in a deterioration of mood. One of our patients, a 34-year-old bookkeeper named Georgia, noticed that for several consecutive winters she had suffered from moodiness, fatigue, and increased appetite. Because she worked for a mail-order house specializing in Christmas decorations and gift items, she attributed the symptoms to an increase in job stress that naturally occurred during the company's busy season. In conversation, however, it emerged that a few years earlier her company's headquarters had been remodeled and she had been moved from her position near a window to an internal office. She often left her house for work before the sun was up, and would leave work long after the sun had gone down. As she realized after a course of phototherapy, "I guess I just haven't been getting my minimum daily requirement of sunlight."

One final example: Howard, a creative director for an advertising agency, began to worry about his ability to hold down a job during his bouts of seasonal depression. Each winter he found it harder and harder to work creatively and efficiently in his high-pressure position. "Normally," he said, "I can look at a piece of artwork and know immediately if it's right. But in the winter I agonize over every little detail. 'Is the color okay? Should this line be thicker, or tilted a little more? Maybe the margin should be wider?' I drive myself and everyone around me totally wacko. Sometimes my inability to move quickly gets me into trouble with other people who have deadlines to meet. I wonder how much longer I'll last in this position."

Nearly 90 out of 100 SAD patients report that they suffer significant disability at work during the winter months, with the universal complaint an inability to concentrate. As illustrated by the preceding anecdotes, other symptoms include difficulty making decisions, a reduction in creative energy and interest in work, reduced output, and problems in working with other people. In addition, SAD can lead to an increase in absenteeism due to illness. Symptoms such as excessive daytime sleepiness constitute a hazard in the workplace that can lead to accidents, endangering not only the patient but coworkers as well. A significant number of patients reported angrily that their seasonal depression had forced them quit their jobs or change careers, as we saw earlier in Nat's case.

Impact on Social Relationships

In our conversations, many SAD patients remark how difficult it is to maintain friendships and meet social obligations during the dark months. Typical of the problem is the experience of Irene, an attractive 29-year-old bank loan officer. Irene says that in the summer her life is filled wth "dancing, dining, and dating," and that she has no trouble in finding male companionship. In the fall, however, her mood begins to change; her relationships likewise begin to crumble. Her feelings of winter depression—hard enough to endure—are only made worse by the acute loneliness she suffers.

Earlier we saw how children and adolescents with SAD experienced social disruption, which often took the form of uncontrollable urges to fight with their schoolmates. Although we ourselves do not see children in our practice at Fair Oaks, (however, there are child psychiatrists on our staff who do treat children and adolescents) the medical literature reports that withdrawal from social activities is a common finding among young people with SAD. Adolescents who enjoy participating on the swim team or in a baseball league during the summer may find that in the winter they pursue such solitary pursuits as reading or video games. For young people with SAD the seasonal change from being active and gregarious to being passive and lonely is not merely a byproduct of the emotional instability of adolescence. It is triggered by the body's response to the amount of light available over the course of the day.

In chapter 6 we will see how phototherapy can be valuable to virtually all patients who meet the criteria for the diagnosis of SAD. As should be clear from these patient stories, however, this disorder, like many illnesses, has an impact not just on the lives of the individuals affected but on their family and social structures as well. In Chapter 7 we will describe how a multifaceted approach to therapy may have the best chance at bringing about improvement in the patient's condition in all its aspects. Such an approach may involve the use of lights, but can also incorporate psychotherapy, family and marital therapy, nutritional counseling, and vocational counseling, as appropriate for the individual patient.

In the next chapter we'll take a close look at the biological reasons underlying SAD and the havoc it wreaks on the mind and body.

Chapter 3

THE CAUSES OF SAD

The hallmark of Seasonal Affective Disorder is its connection to the cycle of seasons. As we have mentioned, light is one of the primary cues your body needs to operate at peak efficiency. Due to some form of biological malfunctioning, patients with SAD are extremely sensitive to the amount of light they receive during the day. If these people aren't exposed to adequate light, or if the light is received at the wrong times, then a number of their body systems begin to operate "out of synch" with one another. Like members of an orchestra who fail to follow the conductor's signals, the organs, glands, and tissues responsible for secreting hormones and other chemicals fall out of harmony with one another. The resulting chemical imbalances produce the symptoms we associate with SAD—symptoms that range from change in appetite to mood swings.

As winter appears, the days grow shorter. Many people rise in darkness, spend their days working in enclosed environments under artificial light, and return to their homes in darkness. In our modern age, it is entirely possible that a typical urban office worker avoids exposure to natural sunlight for weeks, even months at a stretch. For most of us, this presents no serious problem. For patients with SAD, however, the diminishing supply of light throws their whole being into turmoil. Shakespeare's phrase, "The winter of our discontent," holds particular meaning for the patient with SAD.

In addition to seasons, other factors affect the amount of our exposure to light as well. As we discussed in the previous chapter, the latitude at which we live determines the length of our days. For people with SAD, however, a string of three cloudy days in July—even *one* cloudy day, for that matter—can pose a threat.

As we saw in Jenny's case in Chapter 1, when the days begin to shorten at the end of August, patients with SAD generally feel a vague sense of dread or anxiety about the coming winter. During the early fall, this feeling gives way to other symptoms: a slowing down of activity, changes in sleep patterns, and an increased appetite, especially for carbohydrates. By November, the change in a person's affect—the psychiatrist's technical term for mood, emotions, or feelings—is apparent. Patients become sad, sometimes to the point of tears. Their ability to think creatively or to concentrate on work diminishes. They withdraw from family and friends, a situation that can persist up to the onset of spring; the average length of depression in SAD is over five months. Eventually, with increasing daylight, patients begin to feel less depressed and more energetic; their sleep patterns and their appetites also return to normal.

Within just the past few decades, scientists have become increasingly aware of the ubiquity—and importance—of our inner biological rhythms. Rhythms that operate on a daily cycle are called *circadian* (from the Latin "circa," meaning "about," and "dia," meaning "a day"). Circadian rhythms govern most of our body's processes; physical activity, sleep, intake of food and water, body temperature, and the secretion of life-regulating hormones, enzymes, and neurotransmitters.

In order to maintain our health, these rhythms must become synchronized so that they can work together. One of the ways they do so is through exposure to light. The effectiveness of light therapy in treating SAD appears to be related to its role in orchestrating certain circadian rhythms, particularly the rhythm that governs production of a hormone called melatonin, which is secreted by the pineal gland in the brain. We'll discuss this powerful chemical more thoroughly later in this chapter.

SEASONALITY AND BODY RHYTHMS

Animals and humans alike are exquisitely attuned to their environments in ways we are only just beginning to realize. Basic body functions ranging from eating to reproduction are governed by daily and seasonal cycles. As a rule, animals follow a pattern in which their appetites increase in summer, allowing them to accumulate reserves of body fat by fall. Their appetite decreases in winter, corresponding to a drop in the available food supply.

Many animals, including goats, ferrets, horses, mink, and deer, can only conceive offspring at certain times of year. The fact that reproduction is governed by seasonal rhythms enables members of a species to synchronize their activities with changes in their environment. Sheep, for example, are only fertile in the fall. Thus their lambs will be born in the spring, when plenty of food is available to the nursing dams. Sheep breeders have discovered, however, that they can trick the animals into thinking that winter has arrived by shortening their exposure to light over the course of the day. The artificially shortened day triggers the animal's fertility system and thus enables breeders to increase the birth rate. Researchers have found that with hampsters the opposite is true: By shortening the length of their day, they are able to render the animals infertile.

Although humans are fertile year-round, the birth rate does show some seasonal variation that tends to reach a peak in September. Other seasonal patterns have been noticed in the incidence of first menstruation (menarche), the growth rate of children, death rates, and suicide.

Most of our bodily functions, including physical activity, sleep, food consumption, water intake, and body temperature, operate on the circadian rhythms cycles. It has been found, for example, that brain activity and the levels of chemicals called neurotransmitters, responsible for carrying signals across the tiny gaps between neurons, fluctuate over the course of the day. So, too, do the levels of crucial hormones and enzymes. An emerging field of study known as circadian pharmacology is exploring the relationship between body rhythms and the effects of certain medications, including antidepressants.

As we have seen, the control of these rhythms is in large measure a function of the timing and duration of our exposure to bright light. While the rhythms of some animals can be affected by light equal to only half the amount produced by a full moon, it has been found that in humans, even the amount of light found in a typical indoor setting lacks sufficient power to set our daily biological clocks, a process technically known as entrainment.

Some experts theorize that the human species' relative insensitivity to light was conditioned early on in our evolution as a form of self-protection. With the discovery of fire, followed by our ability to control its use, light became available to us throughout the day and night. Theory has it that our bodies had to learn to distinguish the "artificial" light of torches and campfires from the "natural" bright light of the sun, in order to allow entrainment of our circadian rhythms to occur at certain times of day. In the process, humans have adapted to the use of artificial light while retaining their sensitivity to the natural light-dark cycle.

A cyclical, seasonal pattern in mood disorders was recognized in the days of Hippocrates. Even the word "lunatic" originally reflected the belief that the severity of certain mental disorders was somehow connected to the phases of the moon. Since these early glimmerings, the connection between seasonal changes and health has been carefully documented. We know, for example, that the incidence of depression peaks twice during the year, in spring and in autumn. Such seasonality occurs regardless of whether the depression is mild or severe.

Researchers are beginning to find that the severity of symptoms of depression and other disorders is connected to fluctuations in the rhythms that regulate the body chemicals. These substances in turn are responsible for governing our activities and our moods. One study revealed that certain depressed patients have a defective internal "clock" that tends to run fast. If these people are isolated from time cues, such as daylight and interactions with other people, their bodies will operate on a daily cycle that is considerably shorter than the normal cycle of approximately twenty-five hours or so that most of us experience. Such a pattern helps explain why early morning insomnia is a feature of many forms of depression (though not a symptom associated with SAD).

Interestingly, one therapeutic approach to classic depression involves sleep interruption—waking the patient at a certain point in the early morning hours. The benefits of doing so are striking. Most patients report far fewer symptoms of depression the same morning on which their sleep was interrupted. No other therapy, including antidepressant medication, works so quickly. So profound are the effects of sleep deprivation on the symptoms of depression that we often view such a response as a clear clinical indication that the patient is indeed suffering from the disorder. It must be noted, however, that as a rule, patients dislike this form of treatment. Sleep deprivation is particularly hard on patients with SAD, who experience an overwhelming urge to stay in bed, even though, as we have explained, oversleeping makes them feel worse.

The results of sleep deprivation studies suggest that some critical juncture in the circadian cycle regulating depression occurs during the second half of the night, at least in some patients. If these patients are awakened at some point during these hours, the severity of their symptoms will abate dramatically. Such results support the notion that manipulating the timing of sleep at a critical point in time disrupts the rhythms that govern the symptoms of depression. In fact, many experts are convinced that malfunctions in the phase-cycle of circadian rhythms are not merely symptoms of mental disturbances such as manic-depressive illness, but may actually be causing the disorder in and of themselves. For example, sleep deprivation can precipitate a manic episode in some individuals. Research into the effects of insomnia in causing manic cycles is currently being conducted.

Circadian and seasonal patterns in other illnesses ranging from epilepsy to headache have long been demonstrated. Our experience shows them to be strongly related. It is believed that some types of headache may be triggered by the same rhythmic variations in neurotransmitters that are associated with depression. Also, a form of sleep disturbance occurs when body temperature rhythms fall out of whack. When temperature rises too soon, the natural passage through the various phases of sleep is accelerated, causing the body to awaken before the night is over and before adequate rest has been achieved. On the other hand, if the body temperature cycle is delayed, reaching a peak later in the morning, it can result in excessive sleepiness. Knowing patients' individual circadian patterns—classifying them according to whether their cycles peak earlier or later than normal—may eventually become part of our strategy in diagnosing and treating illness.

In most healthy people, the entrainment of circadian rhythms is probably more dependent on time cues provided by interaction with other people—starting work at nine o'clock in the morning, for example, or eating meals at certain times—than on light. People with SAD, however, are hypersensitive to the amount of light in their environment. Many experts now believe that the depressive symptoms associated with SAD are due to a shift in certain circadian rhythms caused by this hypersensitivity. As the seasons change and the days grow shorter, the rhythms reach their peaks at different times than they do during the summer. Because winter sunrise can occur as much as three hours later than in summer, certain physiological events that occur late at night—secretion of hormones, metabolism, and so on—are also shifted three hours later in the day. One explanation proposed for the hypersomnia associated with SAD is that the rhythm governing the onset of sleep has been pushed to a point several hours later in the night. Naturally, a person with such a rhythm disturbance will find it harder to rise in the morning. This hypersensitivity to changes in season, and the yearly pattern of depression, are the key features of SAD.

To illustrate the pattern, we refer again to Louise, whom we met briefly in Chapter 1. If you recall, every autumn Louise felt the onset of a depression so severe that it drove her to seek psychiatric care. After months of therapy—that is to say, by spring—she felt "cured," so that she terminated her sessions with her psychiatrist, only to repeat the cycle again in the fall.

With patients such as Louise, it is important to determine whether their depression is directly connected to the change of seasons or whether it is a major depressive episode that occurs in a yearly pattern that just happens to coincide with the onset of autumn. One way to tell is that SAD responds to light therapy, while other forms of depression do not.

LIGHT, MELATONIN, AND THE BRAIN

How is it that light can have such a powerful effect on the body? By what pathway is the presence of light communicated between the eyes and the brain, triggering the cascade of chemical reactions that helps us maintain our biological equilibrium? More to the point, what aspect of this system is so delicate that the seasonal change in light can disrupt its operations, causing such enormous alterations in mood, appetite, and sleep patterns? What, specifically, causes SAD?

Research into these questions is continuing at centers across America and throughout the world. The results are sometimes conflicting and therefore somewhat confusing. Some evidence suggests, however, that a little-understood brain chemical, a hormone called melatonin, may play some role in the process.

In animals, cycles of fertility and reproduction are rigidly controlled by circadian rhythms, especially the rhythm that governs secretion of melatonin. In contrast, human biological rhythms were thought—until recently, anyway—to be regulated primarily by social and environmental cues. Human activity, including sexual activity, was assumed to be under psychological control, not governed by uncontrollable physical rhythms.

However, in the early 1980s a researcher at the NIMH, Dr. Alfred Lewy, made the pivotal discovery that melatonin secretion by tissues within the brains of both humans and animals is controlled by the amount and timing of light. Lewy's breakthrough was significant because it established a heretofore overlooked continuity between animal and human physiology. Over the past decade we have begun to realize the powerful influence such inborn rhythms can have over virtually every aspect of our functioning. The significance for the field of medicine alone is profound.

As we have seen, the circadian rhythms of human beings require brighter light in order to achieve entrainment than do those of other animals. A light level equal to ordinary room light, for instance, does not affect the rhythms of humans; moonlight, however, is sufficient to affect the rhythms of animals.

Bright light suppresses melatonin secretion; darkness allows melatonin to be produced. Melatonin may be one link in the chain of biological events that govern the regulation of mood, and Lewy's pioneering discovery led to the concept that light might have application as a treatment for depression. At this writing, however, the role of melatonin in affective disorders is still a subject for debate, as we'll see shortly. There is no doubt, however, about the efficacy of light in the treatment of SAD.

The connection between light and neurochemistry is fascinating and complex. It begins when light strikes the eye. Much of the information communicated by light travels to the visual centers of the brain and allows us to see and react to our environment. But some of the information is communicated by a separate pathway that in a sense runs parallel to the optic nerves. These signals are transmitted from the retina directly to the hypothalamus. This cluster of nerves within the brain activates and coordinates a number of basic body functions needed to sustain life: intake of food and water, sleep, and so on. But the hypothalamus is also a crucial part of the limbic system, a group of structures in the brain that regulates moods and emotions, including anger, fear, and sexual arousal.

When activated, the hypothalamus performs a number of tasks. It releases a barrage of chemicals that regulate the function of other glands, especially the pituitary. The pituitary in turn releases a number of important hormones that serve to control the operation of the thyroid, gonads, and adrenal glands perched atop the kidneys. This latter network is sometimes known by the tongue-twisting term the hypothalamic-pituitary-adrenal (HPA) axis. There are other such axes as well: One connects the hypothalamus and the pituitary to the thyroid gland; another connects them to the gonads.

In some people, these axes have been found to be overactive. For some reason, these people have a faulty biological "thermostat" that is supposed to regulate and give feedback to the glands and thus put the brakes on the production of chemicals. As a result too many chemicals are released. For example, one consequence of a malfunction in the HPA axis is that the adrenal glands produce excessive quantities of substances called corticosteroids.

As we mentioned, some of the signals from the retina can trigger visual signals, so that we perceive objects in our environment. Other signals stimulate activity along the various hypothalamic axes. And another group of the retinal signals is transmitted along yet another pathway. These signals travel through the optic nerve to the hypothalamus and then to another organ within the brain, the pineal gland, one function of which, some experts believe, is to help us adapt to changes in our environment. When the pineal gland is stimulated by a substance called noradrenaline, a hormone, melatonin, is produced and secreted. (We should also note that production of melatonin is also controlled to some extent by signals from superior cervical ganglia, a part of the nervous system located in the spinal cord.)

Secretion of this powerful hormone occurs largely at night. In other words, as long as light of a certain intensity is present, signals traveling from the retina through the hypothalamus to the pineal *prevent* the production of melatonin. As Dr. Lewy discovered, once those signals have been switched off, melatonin production begins.

Advances in diagnostic technology have allowed physicians to examine the blood levels of such hormones as melatonin with remarkable accuracy. We can now monitor such levels to find clues that indicate how well the organs along the hypothalamic axes are functioning. In a sense, these hormones offer us a window on the brain. Finding abnormal levels of melatonin or an abnormal timing of secretion, for example, might lead us to investigate whether the hypothalamus is not working in other ways as well. And because one malfunctioning gland affects the functions of all the other glands connected to it along the various axes, the combined disruptions in function can snowball and result in a number of illnesses, of which depression is one.

MELATONIN

As we indicated, the primary function of melatonin in animals appears to be the regulation and coordination of seasonal reproductive cycles, so that births occur during the most advantageous time of the year to guarantee survival of the offspring. In humans, however, its effect on the reproductive system is less clear. Some researchers believe melatonin inhibits ovulation and modifies the secretion of other substances by a number of other glands. Melatonin in humans may affect the release by the pituitary of a number of hormones, including luteinizing hormone (involved in ovulation and secretion of estrogen), prolactin (which stimulates milk production), follicle-stimulating hormone (which stimulates maturation of the ovary and the production of sperm cells in the male), thyroid-stimulating hormone, and perhaps others as well.

Melatonin levels change dramatically over time. In the course of a single twenty-four-hour period, for example, the nighttime level can rise anywhere from two to twenty times as high as the daytime level. Such fluctuation poses problems for the physician trying to establish a patient's "normal" melatonin levels; obviously, one's melatonin level relates directly to the time of day at which a reading is taken.

Interestingly, the body seems to manufacture melatonin as a kind of natural sleeping pill. As we have seen, during the course of the night, we progress through the various stages of sleep. After the rapid-eye movement (REM or dream sleep) stage, our sleep quickly becomes lighter, culminating in a brief period of arousal before we fall back asleep and begin the cycle over again. Interestingly, research indicates that during these brief arousals the body increases its production of melatonin, perhaps as a way of helping us fall asleep again. By the same token, melatonin secretion has been found to be at its low point during REM sleep.

The connection between mental illness and brain chemicals has been recognized for some time. Abnormal levels of such neurotransmitters as serotonin, norepinephrine, and acetylcholine, for example, are associated with the presence of depressive illness. Interestingly, these same chemicals are involved in the process of melatonin synthesis.

Some individuals who attempt suicide have significantly higher melatonin levels than other people. Other evidence suggests that melatonin secretion can be permanently influenced by emotional trauma at crucial stages of development. For example, a study revealed that adults who had experienced loss of their parents before age 17 had subnormal levels of melatonin. The lowest levels were found in those patients whose parents died during the first years of the patients' lives. Such findings suggest that the body's mechanism for synthesizing melatonin may be disrupted by emotional shock especially at an early stage of development. Abnormal serotonin levels are also considered to be a sign of suicide risk. Further research may indicate to what extent the level of melatonin production is determined by an individual's genetic inheritance.

Recently, researchers have found that melatonin levels are abnormally increased in people with manic disorders, and are abnormally low in people with some kinds of depression. There is, in fact, a "low melatonin syndrome" in depression. The syndrome is characterized by low melatonin levels, abnormal findings during certain diagnostic tests for depression, and disturbed circadian rhythms in the production of a substance called cortisol, a corticosteroid produced by the adrenal gland and part of the hypothalamic-pituitary-adrenal axis. It also appears that depressed patients with low melatonin exhibit less variation in their symptoms during the day as well as over the course of a year.

As you can see, some evidence seems to suggest that increased secretion of melatonin is one mechanism that produces sleepiness, irritability, social withdrawal, and depression—the main symptoms of SAD. At this point, however, researchers are not absolutely certain whether melatonin is directly involved in causing SAD, or whether abnormalities in melatonin secretion are simply a by-product, or a "marker," of the illness. Some experts suspect that exposure to light has a general impact on the complex biochemistry of the brain, perhaps resulting in an increased concentration of other neurotransmitters such as serotonin, which in turn can affect the level of melatonin in the body. Resolution of many of these uncertainties awaits further research. At this point, however, let's look at some of the issues involved and the discoveries made thus far.

LIGHT, MELATONIN, AND SAD

The effect of light on mood has long been recognized by the medical profession. As long ago as 1898, for example, a doctor named Frederick Cook, who participated in an expedition into the Antarctic, found that artificial bright light improved the condition of members of the ship's crew who had become affected, "body and soul, with languor" during the long polar winter.

Not until the early 1980s, however, did the use of light as therapy become a recognized technique. The pioneer in this field is Dr. Norman Rosenthal, a colleague of Dr. Lewy's at the

National Institute of Mental Health. Dr. Rosenthal was aware that melatonin produces seasonal changes in the behavior of many different animals. Because SAD is also seasonal in nature, he began to wonder if melatonin might play some role in the onset and severity of the disorder.

Following Dr. Lewy's discovery of the suppressive effect of light on melatonin secretion, Dr. Rosenthal wondered what would happen if patients with SAD were exposed to bright light during their depressive periods. Indeed, he found that the impact of light—the rapidity and thoroughness with which it relieves SAD symptoms—was dramatic. Although research into the subject is by no means complete, one explanation for the effect of light on SAD is that it helps to set the biological clock that governs the secretion of melatonin (and perhaps other rhythms as well). Subsequent research has shown that, indeed, there is a subgroup of SAD patients who have melatonin rhythms that are significantly delayed compared to normal patients, and that bright light advances the time of onset of melatonin secretion. Again we must stress that an abnormal melatonin rhythm is not necessarily the cause of depressive symptoms; it is merely one detectable sign that the brain structures responsible for regulating such rhythms are out of whack.

In some patients with manic-depressive disorders, melotonin secretion can be suppressed up to 50 percent by light measured at 500 lux. In comparison, ordinary indoor light usually ranges from 100 to 300 lux; the light used in SAD therapy is much brighter, ranging from 2,000 to 10,000 lux.

Other factors besides light affect melatonin levels in the body. Research is under way to test the hypothesis that consumption of carbohydrates affects the synthesis of neurotransmitters and their various intermediate forms. However, we have not found a purely dietary approach to handling the symptoms of SAD to be of any value.

Not all experts on SAD agree that the level of melatonin and its rhythm of secretion lie at the root of the problem. For these researchers, evidence is not conclusive that suppression of melatonin secretion, by light or any other means, directcy produces antidepressant effects. In one experiment patients were given atenolol, a medication classified as a beta-blocker. Drugs of this category are known to interfere with the secretion of melatonin. Theoretically this technique should have produced the same antidepressant effect as phototherapy, since both strategies suppress melatonin secretion. While beta-blockers did decrease melatonin levels, no antidepressant effect was seen.

It's possible that the problem lies not in the levels of melatonin but in the heightened sensitivity of melatonin receptors in the organs and tissues of a particular person's body. Furthermore, some studies have tested the effects of different levels of light. In one such study, light exposure that had no apparent effect on melatonin secretion produced as much relief from SAD symptoms as brighter light that did suppress melatonin.

One way researchers assess the relationship between light and melatonin has been to administer doses of pure melatonin and see whether such increased levels of the hormone will offset the beneficial effects of light. In a number of studies, giving oral melatonin has indeed been found to reintroduce some of the symptoms light therapy had relieved: hypersomnia, overeating, cravings for carbohydrates. Such symptoms, however, did not translate into significantly increased feelings of depression on standardized depression rating scales. In very large quantities, doses of melatonin can trigger depressive symptoms in people who have already been diagnosed as depressed. Oral melatonin has also been found to have a tranquilizing effect. In one study, melatonin administered by injection or as a nasal spray was found to induce sleep.

As should be clear from this discussion, the role of melatonin in SAD is not yet fully known. However, research on melatonin extended our understanding of the degree that both human and animal physiology is under the control of circadian rhythms, and that these rhythms in turn are regulated by exposure to light. This in turn was the key discovery that led to the development of phototherapy. Exactly what role is played by a particular rhythm, such as the rhythm of melatonin, in the development of SAD is an open question and is currently the focus of much debate among professionals concerned with treating patients who suffer from the disorder. Further studies will help clarify our picture of the role of melatonin in regulating mood. However, as with much scientific study, the answer to one question will stimulate dozens of others; the more we know about the way the body works, the more we realize how complex and interdependent its systems are.

OTHER FACTORS

Melatonin is only one of many substances that act and interact with each other to produce neural responses in our bodies and that regulate every aspect of their function. In fact, melatonin is actually the final product in a series of processes involved in the metabolism of certain amino acids. At this point, then, we should touch on some of the other substances that are involved in the complex neural network and that may play a role in the development—and treatment—of Seasonal Affective Disorder.

One such substance is the amino acid called tryptophan, found in certain protein-rich foods such as milk, liver, lean meats, poultry, peanut butter, and legumes. Tryptophan is a *precursor* of serotonin; a precursor is a substance from which another, often more active, substance is formed. When metabolized during the process of digestion, tryptophan helps supply niacin, a nutrient that helps process the sugars needed to create the nucleic acids found in every cell of the body. Evidence suggests that tryptophan undergoes significant seasonal fluctuation; the level of tryptophan found in the serum as well as the total amount of tryptophan in the body vary over the course of a year.

For some people tryptophan can have a sedative effect; many people, in fact, consume large doses of tryptophan purchased as a nutritional supplement at health-food stores in an effort to improve the speed with which they fall asleep. At Fair Oaks we sometimes recommend the use of tryptophan to patients with sleep difficulties.

In addition, some evidence suggests that tryptophan may enhance the antidepressant effects of certain medications in patients who do not respond to therapy with a single antidepressant. This notion sprang from the fact that tryptophan is converted by the body into serotonin. Serotonin is primarily a neurotransmitter that helps transmit signals across the gaps between nerves in the brain, but it performs other crucial functions as well. In humans, serotonin inhibits the secretion of stomach acids and other digestive juices, constricts blood vessels, stimulates certain muscles, and helps transmit signals across the gaps between nerves in the brain. Significantly, depressed people are known to lack adequate levels of serotonin. Thus consuming foods with tryptophan means more serotonin will be produced to augment the antidepressant effects of medications working on the mood-controlling serotonin systems of the brain.

Among psychiatrists, the use of tryptophan to enhance therapy with medications—a technique known as "precursor loading" —has dropped off in recent years. For one thing, tryptophan must be given in very high doses in order to produce its effects. However, there is an emerging trend toward a more naturalistic approach to healing in many medical disciplines, including psychiatry. Perhaps, like many things, treatment strategies run in cycles, and in the near future we'll see a resurgence of interest in such approaches.

Not surprisingly, serotonin, like its chemical "parent" tryptophan, shows significant seasonal variation, not only in the levels found in platelets but in the ability of the body to absorb and use it. One study—the first to demonstrate pronounced seasonal rhythms in the chemicals of the central nervous system—showed that the amount of serotonin found in the hypothalamus was highest in late autumn, but reached a low point during December and January. The investigators concluded that seasonal rhythms in the human brain, spinal fluid, and blood components exist; what's more, these rhythms are of considerable magnitude.

Also, intake of carbohydrates can accelerate the metabolism of serotonin. The process is roughly as follows: Intake of carbohydrate-rich foods triggers the release of insulin, which is used to break down the sugars contained in carbohydrates. The presence of insulin in turn accelerates the brain's ability to absorb tryptophan, which stimulates synthesis of serotonin. Since serotonin helps relieve depression, some experts think that people who consume enormous quantities of carbohydrates are actually helping themselves by replenishing their supplies of serotonin—or eventually, perhaps, of melatonin, which is the substance that results when serotonin is acted on by enzymes.

As we mentioned, cortisol is a glucocorticoid produced by the adrenal glands in response to stress. In normal people, the serum level of cortisol usually falls off in late evening. However, a study of healthy people in Norway found that, during the long dark autumn and winter at that latitude, their bodies increased the production and concentration of cortisol. One conclusion that can be drawn from such findings is that prolonged darkness is stressful, even for normal individuals, and that the body must compensate by producing chemicals to offset its impact. We mentioned these findings to illustrate the fact that all types of bodily substances—hormones, neurotransmitters, steroids—have been found to demonstrate circadian rhythmicity, as well as seasonal variation. It may turn out that any or all of them are involved in triggering Seasonal Affective Disorder.

Chapter 4

SAD AND OTHER MENTAL DISORDERS

For nearly a decade Mark, a construction worker, experienced bouts of moodiness, loss of energy, and changes in eating habits that followed a yearly cycle—worse in the winter, better in spring and summer. In an effort to find relief, Mark had seen several doctors, each of whom, it seemed, gave his illness a different name: hypothyroidism; hypoglycemia; depression. None of the medications they prescribed, however, helped to improve his condition significantly.

Mark came to Fair Oaks in the winter of 1987. After hearing his story and conducting a thorough physical and mental examination, we told Mark we suspected he was suffering from Seasonal Affective Disorder. As we described the illness to him, he nodded his head. "This is it," he interjected a number of times.

Following a regimen of phototherapy, used in combination with a carefully monitored course of antidepressant medications, many of Mark's symptoms abated. Naturally he was happy to find effective relief after all those years of suffering. But just as important, he said, was the fact that his illness had finally been given the right name. As he put it, "It's such a relief just knowing that other people recognize this disease exists, and that it's not just something I made up in my head."

For Mark, and for many other SAD patients, giving their

enemy a name is the first step—and in some ways, perhaps, the most critical step—in conquering the disorder.

Effective medical treatment begins with an accurate diagnosis. Obviously, a problem cannot be solved until it has been identified. Only then can a remedy be selected that has a chance of being effective.

At this point we should stress that our intention in the following pages is simply to inform you of some of the steps a qualified physician takes in arriving at a diagnosis. The information we present is not intended to substitute for medical analysis by a professional. If you or someone you know is suffering from signs of depression, or any other illness for that matter, we cannot emphasize strongly enough the fact that you should place yourself in the hands of a doctor who can order the proper tests needed to reveal the true nature of your problem. By the same token, you should not undertake any of the therapeutic strategies we mention without the guidance of a medical professional.

Fortunately, the work of many skillful and dedicated researchers in recent years has made it easier for patients with SAD to be diagnosed and treated. Studies involving hundreds of patients have served to identify both the disease and its pattern of symptoms. And the recognition of SAD as an "official" diagnosis means that more and more physicians will eventually be able to spot the condition and offer relief to their patients.

Despite these advances, however, a diagnosis of SAD can be an elusive goal. For one thing, its seasonal pattern means that symptoms appear only over the course of a year—a significantly long period of time. Many people who suffer a bout of depression in the winter might dismiss it as "cabin fever" or "holiday blues" or some other mild, transient condition. When their depression occurs again the following year, they may have forgotten what had happened many months before. Only if the pattern persists, year after year, do they begin to realize that they suffer from a truly seasonal illness. Indeed, one criterion for determining the presence of SAD is that the condition has existed for at least two years out of the last three. Diseases with such long cycles are difficult for patients, as well as physicians, to perceive.

In many cases the symptoms of the disorder are not so devastating or life-threatening that people feel they must seek immediate help. They often feel they can "ride it out" until the spring, coping with depleted energy or moodiness as best they can. Such resistance is certainly understandable. Getting medical help is costly and time-consuming. Some people, like Mark, who have sought help only to be given a wrong diagnosis or inappropriate therapy, find that no one can help them using traditional approaches to depression; their confidence in doctors has been undermined. In addition, people fear that being diagnosed with a mental illness could have serious ramifications on their lives at home, in the workplace, and in society as a whole.

Another complicating factor is that SAD, like many serious psychiatric disorders, is not a single problem but a syndrome of multiple symptoms that can sometimes confuse the clinical picture. In some cases patients experience changes in their patterns of appetite or sleep and are referred to Fair Oaks specifically for treatment of an "eating disorder" or a "sleeping disorder." We may find, however, that these symptoms are a part of a broader clinical picture. Other patients might present a long list of different complaints. It takes a certain degree of perseverance—not to mention skill—to resist seeing each of these complaints as a discrete psychological problem, and to see instead the broader picture that unites the multiple symptoms into a single, unified diagnosis.

Given these obstacles, how does the physician arrive at a diagnosis of SAD?

SAD: MEETING THE CRITERIA

In order for SAD to be recognized, the psychiatrist must consider and rule out other types of disorders, both organic and psychiatric. There is of course more to it. Before diagnosis can be confirmed, a patient must fulfill certain other specific criteria. As with any illness, these criteria are important in helping identify the specific problem confronting the treating physician. If no clear guidelines exist, the illness may not be recognized or may be misidentified. The consequences of such an error—placing the patient under therapy that is at best ineffective and at worst dangerous—can be serious.

Fortunately, a patient with SAD usually demonstrates a recognizable pattern of symptoms that have been identified, agreed on, and refined by SAD researchers over the past few years. According to the DSM-III-R, the diagnostic criteria for SAD are as follows:

1. The patient has symptoms of a major depression that meets the definition accepted by the medical profession.
2. Other primary physical illnesses can definitely be ruled out as a factor in initiating and maintaining the mood disturbance.
3. The patient exhibits certain patterns of associated symptoms, including hypersomnia, increased appetite, weight gain, and/or fatigue.
4. The depression exhibits a certain seasonal pattern:
   - The symptoms occur during a particular 60-day period of the year (for example, between the beginning of October and the end of November).
   - The depression also disappears during a particular 60-day period (for example, between mid-February and mid-April).
   - An episode of disturbed mood that follows this seasonal pattern occurs at least once a year for three different years; two of those years must be consecutive.
   - The depression occurs during a sustained two-week period over which the symptoms occur nearly every day.
   - The depressive symptoms are not related to some obvious seasonal stress, such as being unemployed every winter or having negative associations with certain holidays.

- Seasonal episodes of mood disturbance outnumber any nonseasonal episodes by at least three to one.

Let's look at each of these points in detail.

According to the first criterion, a patient with SAD must demonstrate, to a certain level, the recognizable pattern of symptoms of depression: slowed thinking, decreased pleasure and activity, feelings of guilt and hopelessness, and abnormal patterns of sleeping and eating. The DSM-III-R provides a complete list of these symptoms.

Once depression has been identified, it is further classified according to severity, patterns of recurrence, and whether or not episodes alternate with times when mood is abnormally elevated. In most cases of SAD, patients suffer from depression of mild to moderate severity. Indeed many people with SAD do experience elevated moods in the spring, when the days begin to grow longer. As we have seen, though, the main thing that distinguishes SAD from other types of depression is its distinctive annual cycle. The symptoms of fatigue, moodiness, and appetite changes appear during the winter months, when days are shorter and exposure to natural light is limited. The presence of such a pattern over a period of at least two years fulfills part of the fourth criterion for SAD. (Keep in mind, however, that the absence of sunlight during any part of the year can cause a SAD patient to experience a bout of depression.)

We should note that, despite its good intentions, the DSM-III-R has many flaws. Diagnosing depression through a list of clinical symptoms can lead even thoughtful psychiatrists to overlook the true nature and cause of illness. For one thing, symptoms can be highly subjective: Two different patients might describe the same complaint in a completely different way.

Furthermore, the manual gives no guidance to the dozens of organic conditions, ranging from endocrine disorders to nutritional deficiencies, that can cause symptoms of depression. Yet to provide the best care for our patients, we as psychiatrists must look beyond the surface in order to determine exactly what is happening inside the patient's mind and body. To do so, and to meet the second SAD criterion, we must consider whether the patient is suffering from an organic illness. In many cases, careful history taking and laboratory testing will reveal the reasons for the patient's suffering. Lab tests in particular are not discussed in DSM-III-R.

In one sense, depression might be thought of as a "physical" illness, in that it usually arises from a malfunction in brain chemistry. Strictly speaking, however, the precise pathophysiology of SAD is unknown. In diagnosing the condition it is crucial to search for, and rule out, any organic illness that might be held responsible for causing the symptoms of depression and that can be treated separately. If such an illness can be found, that illness is considered to be primary, and the symptoms of depression that result are secondary in nature. SAD, on the other hand, produces primary depression.

One of the interesting features of SAD is that, while it does produce certain changes in mood and mental ability that classify it as a form of depression, it also produces other symptoms that, until recently, were thought to be the mirror image of depression. For example, patients with what has been considered "classic" depression suffer from diminished appetite, weight loss, and a certain pattern of insomnia (early morning wakening). SAD patients, on the other hand, have greater appetites, gain weight, and sleep more than usual. Thus these symptoms were at one time said to be "atypical" because they were not thought to be typical of the severe depression usually encountered in psychiatric practice. It is now realized, however, that such symptoms are more commonly present, and thus they are included as part of the description of a major depressive episode. If a patient demonstrates these symptoms, the third criterion for diagnosing SAD has been met.

Because of the unique characteristics of SAD, the standard tests given to assess the level of depression in a particular patient may be inadequate, at least to a certain degree. As a result, supplemental surveys may be needed to evaluate the impact of the disorder on the patient. SAD's demonstrable connection to the seasons, for example, is not generally a feature of typical depression, and can be analyzed separately. The atypical nature of the disorder also suggests that SAD patients are *biologically* different from patients with other forms of depression. Research is being conducted to identify exactly what those physical differences might be, and how they might affect the course of therapy.

The last criterion helps define the "seasonal" aspect of Seasonal Affective Disorder. Such a precise definition helps to rule out any depressive episodes that just happen to occur during the winter but which are not directly related to the change of seasons and which do not recur on an annual basis.

There are exceptions to this pattern of symptoms typically associated with SAD. Some SAD patients experience winter depressions but do not exhibit abnormally elevated mood in the summer. Their disorder is thus said to be unipolar in nature, whereas some SAD patients experience mania. Approximately seven percent of SAD patients do have episodes of extreme mood elevations—mania—during the summer months. And as we will see, there are variations in which certain patients experience some, but not all, of the SAD symptoms, while others experience depression during the summertime and elevated mood in the winter, a condition that has come to be known as "reverse SAD."

Although SAD has only been recognized for a few years, there is already evidence of a long-term pattern to the illness. As a rule, patients begin to notice winter depression in late adolescence; each year the depression grows progressively worse as they reach their mid-twenties. At this point we are not certain whether the disorder continues to grow in severity as the years pass, or whether it reaches a plateau.

Despite the recent recognition of SAD as a specific disorder, and despite the clear evidence that SAD patients respond to light therapy whereas those with other types of depression do not, there are some physicians who are still reluctant to consider SAD as a potential diagnosis. They do not feel the evidence accumulated thus far indicates that SAD is a distinct subtype of depression. At worst, such professional skepticism may prevent some patients from finding the help they need to remedy their problem. On the brighter side, however, skepticism prompts researchers to conduct more studies and to analyze their data even more carefully in order to refine understanding of this disorder.

SAD, DEPRESSION, AND OTHER TYPES OF MENTAL ILLNESS

Depression is a complex problem. Feelings of sadness, despair, or discouragement are a natural, indeed normal, reaction to stress, bereavement, or disappointment. All of us at one time or another complain of being "down in the dumps" or having "the blues." A previously active, healthy woman who suffers a broken hip and who can no longer walk out of her house to visit friends may begin to experience a very real form of depression. Usually, though, when the situation that triggers unhappiness is over—when we find that new job, or pass the final exam, or regain our health—the depression lifts and our mood improves.

In other cases, symptoms of depression represent not a disorder of their own, but rather a sign that some other underlying physical or mental problem exists. There are over 75 organic diseases, ranging from cancer and heart disease to infectious mononucleosis and hepatitis, that can produce some of the symptoms associated with depression. Similarly, certain other types of mental illness can trick the unwary physician into using the catch-all diagnosis of depression and thus prescribing the wrong treatment.

For some people, however, depression is a specific mental illness in and of itself, one of a category of psychiatric illnesses called mood disorders.

Clinically speaking, a mood is a prolonged emotional state that affects every aspect of a person's life. Moods can be high, low, or somewhere in between. It should be noted that mood disorders are different entities entirely from psychotic illnesses such as schizophrenia or delusional disorders.

A low mood, of course, is called depression. A very elevated mood is known as mania, and is characterized by high levels of energy, rapid speech, and sometimes by grandiose notions of self-importance. Somewhere between these extremes lies *hypomania*. Hypomania is a psychopathologic state, an abnormality of mood that is higher than normal euphoria but not as high as mania. It is further characterized by feelings of expansiveness, unrealistic optimism, rapid speech and activity, and a decreased need for sleep. While some hypomanic patients experience increased periods of creativity during these periods, others may show irritability, poor judgment, or flashes of anger. A patient suffering from a hypomanic episode will not experience hallucinations. Hypomania is not severe enough to cause marked impairment in the ability to function at work or in society, nor does it require hospitalization. It does, however, require medical attention. The patient must be observed carefully so that any progression of the condition can be noted. If a patient is under phototherapy and his hypomania persists, then the dosage of light must be reduced and perhaps discontinued. If the mood elevation continues to the point where it crosses over into mania, treatment with lithium would be considered.

There are two main types of mood disorders: depressive and bipolar. The term "bipolar" refers to the fact that the patient's mood swings between two poles, or extremes, that represent either end of the emotional spectrum.

Depressive disorders are illnesses in which the patient suffers one or more periods of depression without experiencing the swing into a manic or hypomanic state. One type of depressive disorder is known as major depression, and is the condition most people think of when they use the general term "depression." It is the most common adult psychiatric disorder: As many as fifteen out of every hundred people experience a depressive episode at some point in their lives.

Bipolar disorders are further broken down into two types, depending on the range of the mood swing experienced by the patient. Bipolar I disorders are those in which the patient alternates between periods of extremely elevated mood (mania) and extremely depressed mood. Manic depression is a bipolar I disorder. Criteria for diagnosing manic episode include an abnormal and persistently elevated, expansive, or irritable mood marked by such symptoms as inflated self-esteem, decreased need for sleep, racing thoughts, easy distractability, and risk-taking behavior. The mood disturbance is severe enough to impair the ability to function and may necessitate hospitalization.

Typically, a manic depressive individual will suffer a number of extreme mood swings (normal to manic to depressed and back to normal) over the course of a lifetime. However, some manic depressives, known as rapid cyclers, might experience as many as four or five such swings each year.

A bipolar II disorder is one in which the mood swing is less extreme than in a bipolar I disorder. The swing ranges from hypomanic to depressed and back again to normal. In other words, the extreme manic component is missing.

SAD is often a bipolar II disorder. Many SAD patients in the United States demonstrate a lifelong history of bipolar II illness; the incidence of bipolar disorders with SAD varies in other countries. Simply put, SAD patients feel depressed in the winter and normally happy in the summer. In some cases, however, the happiness is actually "too happy" to be considered appropriate, at which point it is considered to be hypomania. By defining the condition carefully, physicians are able to distinguish SAD from manic depression, a condition that requires a different approach to treatment.

At this point we should note that bipolar II disorders are sometimes confused with another type of mental illness known as borderline personality disorder. Confusion between the two is perhaps understandable, since both types of disorder have certain traits in common.

Patients with borderline personality disorders experience difficulty deciding "who they are"—what career they should follow or which values to adopt. This identity problem often shows as chronic feelings of emptiness or boredom. They also display inappropriate, intense, or uncontrolled anger toward other people. Naturally, such emotions can disrupt relationships with family, friends, and coworkers. Oftentimes a person with a borderline disorder will alternate between feelings of worship or overidealization of another person and total loathing or devaluation. Borderline individuals have difficulty tolerating being alone, and will go to extreme lengths to avoid suffering abandonment, either real or imaginary.

Borderline individuals are prone to instability in their moods. Often this instability appears as shifts from their "normal" disposition to depression, irritability, or anxiety. Such people often exhibit self-destructive tendencies, ranging in severity from reckless driving to suicidal behavior; such actions are often taken in order to manipulate others. If you saw the movie *Fatal Attraction*, you may recognize that the character portrayed by Glenn Close displayed many of these traits.

Volumes could be written about this curious form of mental illness. For our purposes, however, we must limit our discussion to the contrasts between a borderline personality disorder and a bipolar II disorder, specifically SAD. For one thing, while both illnesses can cause extreme changes in behavior, the mood shifts in borderline illness are frequently short-lived, a reaction to stress, and fluctuate between anger, irritability, and depression, whereas the depression of SAD persists for months. While SAD patients may suffer a lack of self-esteem, such feelings can be directly attributed to such real symptoms as weight gain or difficulties in the home or on the job caused by their depressed mood. In borderline disorders, the lack of self-esteem often has no such recognizable cause. Borderline individuals fear abandonment; SAD patients often choose to withdraw from social activities. Lastly, borderline patients attempt to manipulate others into gratifying their needs. While the family and friends of SAD patients may indeed feel manipulated by their loved ones' condition—having to compensate for their lack of energy, forced to feel and act sympathetically for weeks on end—manipulation is not the intent of the patient with SAD.

SAD IS NOT "WINTER BLUES"

At this point we should emphasize that SAD is a recognized mental disorder with a precisely defined list of symptoms. It should not be confused with "holiday blues," those bouts of depression that attack some people around the time of the year-end festivities. For these individuals, the stress and pressure that occurs around Christmas can become overwhelming: The seemingly endless parties, the socializing with people—family and friends—whom they have managed to avoid the rest of the year, are seen as burdensome.

The intense emotional associations with which we imbue our holidays, ranging from nostalgia to dread, can also trigger changes in mood. Many people are haunted by unhappy or traumatic memories from their childhood, memories that are triggered by the sights, sounds, and smells of the holiday. Some of our patients, for example, report that the holidays were bad times where relatives drank more alcohol than usual and would become abusive or violent. Supposedly happy times can become torturous for people who live alone or who have suffered the recent death of a loved one. For many, simply returning to the ordinary routine of January, following the events of the previous month, is depressing.

In contrast, SAD patients may love Christmas but hate winter. The distinction between SAD and holiday blues is illustrated by a comment made by one of our patients. She told us that she cherished the excitement of the holiday but was unable to slough off her seasonal depression in order to participate in family activities. As she put it, "If only Christmas came on the Fourth of July." Another way to recognize SAD is that its symptoms begin in the early fall; holiday blues usually don't show up until after Thanksgiving, when the signs of Christmas—the decorations, the music—become pervasive.

Nor is SAD just another name for the cold-weather mood slumps commonly known as "winter blues" or "winter blahs" or "cabin fever." Those names are often given to the relatively mild, short-lived periods of unhappiness experienced by a large number of otherwise healthy people during the dead of winter. Far from being "mental disorders," cabin fever and its cousins can be thought of in one sense as normal reactions to the restrictions and realities of the cold season. During the winter, of course, we are forced to curtail our warm-weather pattern of activities. It becomes harder to socialize and exercise. Living in enforced proximity with others for extended periods of time can contribute to boredom, fatigue, and a feeling of being closed in. Predictably, if you spend December looking forward to your two-week Caribbean vacation scheduled for February, you may begin to feel a little edgy sometime around the middle of January. The exact nature of "winter blues" is hard to pin down. The experience of such feelings seldom drives sufferers to seek medical attention, and so far there have been no controlled studies that might identify the physical and emotional impact of seasonal changes on a so-called "typical" individual.

SAD does share some traits in common with its milder cousins. They all tend to make people feel bored, edgy, irritable, and cooped-up. Such feelings, naturally, contribute to stress; stress, in turn, can exacerbate depression and can lead to physical problems, such as fatigue, sleep disturbance, or aches and pains. In extreme cases, fortunately rare, people in these circumstances may experience hallucinations or become violent. Actually, violence as a seasonal symptom is more likely to occur during the summer, a phenomenon we'll discuss in more detail in Chapter 5.

There may be another factor at work in triggering the onset of cabin fever. During the winter, it's entirely possible that, as a legacy from our evolutionary past, the inner rhythms that govern our biological functions experience a natural slowing down. In other words, such a reduction in activity and metabolism might have conveyed some sort of survival advantage to our ancestors during the time of year when food and energy were scarce. Now, though, in the age of electric lights and plentiful food, that genetic legacy is perceived as more of a nuisance than an asset. Cabin fever seldom requires medical attention. A change in routine or an increase in the level of exercise may be all that's needed. SAD, however, is different. As Carla Hellekson, a psychiatrist in Fairbanks, Alaska, put it, "SAD is more than the winter blahs. This is something that needs to be taken care of."

Finally, though, the thing that distinguishes SAD from all other forms of depression is the treatment that is used—light—and the response it can produce. Whereas typical depression can be treated effectively through the combined use of antidepressant medication and counseling, such a strategy is usually not completely effective in managing SAD. In our experience, medication used alone failed to produce the desired results in every one of our SAD patients. Similarly, counseling may help patients cope with the effects of SAD on their lives, but will not treat the disorder directly. In patients with clear-cut, classic cases of SAD, the benefits of light therapy—sometimes referred to as phototherapy—are enormous. No other strategy can make such a claim. As one SAD patient told a magazine reporter, her reaction to phototherapy was like "flying high on sunshine."

CHAPTER 5

DIAGNOSING SAD

PATIENT HISTORY

The first step in diagnosing SAD, or indeed any medical disorder, is to obtain a thorough history of the patient's condition. As a rule, the history of a psychiatric illness is harder to trace than that of a physical illness or injury. The clues we gather during this initial conversation alert us to a number of important facts about the illness—not just the overt signs but the more subtle ways the illness is impinging on the patient's life as well. Another resource in this part of the procedure is corroborative information supplied in interviews with the patient's spouse, other relatives, or close friends.

Our overall goal in taking the history is to learn which symptoms the patient identifies as being prominent in his or her condition. Some of the questions we ask are basic: When do you notice your depression coming on? What are the symptoms that drove you to seek medical help? When did you first become aware of your symptoms? What is the first thing you notice when you start to feel depressed? Do you feel worse at any particular time of day? Have you noticed any particular pattern to your symptoms? What events or conflicts seem to trigger or precipitate your depression?

We also inquire about changes in eating or sleeping habits or weight gain, regardless of whether the patient reports having noticed them as symptoms. Oftentimes we find that a period of many months has intervened between the time patients first experience symptoms and when they decide to see a doctor. Many times we find that because of the length of time over which the symptoms may occur, patients have been unaware of many of the changes in their lives until their memories are jogged through the history-taking process.

Of course, as the fourth criterion mentioned in Chapter 4 illustrates, one of the most important aspects of the patient's history of SAD is the seasonal pattern of the illness. Typically the thing that tips us off to the presence of SAD is the patient's remark that he or she "dreads" the time of year when the leaves change. Other patients might comment that in winter all they feel like doing is "hibernating." This undisputed pattern of depression that begins in winter and remits with the arrival of spring is of course the key piece in the SAD jigsaw puzzle.

Another important clue, though, is the pattern of symptoms. While foremost among these is depressed mood, the pattern also usually involves oversleeping, changes in eating habits (specifically carbohydrate cravings and accompanying weight gain), and profound lethargy. The presence of these symptoms helps to differentiate SAD from other types of depression.

Because our psychiatric practices are hospital-based, our patients tend to be more severely depressed than those seen by physicians on an outpatient basis. As a result, the histories of these patients usually reveal a telling clue to the presence of SAD. Specifically, these patients have been treated by a number of physicians prior to their referral to Fair Oaks, and have been given a variety of antidepressant medications over a relatively long period of time. However, they have not responded to these medications as well as would normally be expected. Usually they have been prescribed two or three different standard tricyclic antidepressant medications, the so-called "first-line" medications, yet have failed to show adequate improvement. Many of these patients have even been tried on the "second line" therapies—those medications that work in different ways and pose a somewhat higher risk of side effects, but again show less response than would be expected.

This history of resistance to therapy is a strong tipoff that the depression is anything but typical and may need a different approach to treatment. When we spot a history such as that we've just described, we take particular care to unearth any clues to a seasonal pattern to the patient's symptoms. We may ask point blank, for example, whether the patient has noticed a seasonal pattern to mood changes. If that approach seems too direct, we may inquire whether one time of year seems worse than another. The process of eliciting a history of seasonal depression is a slow one; it may take many questions over many sessions to pin down the true nature of the problem. As we get to know our patients better, we may realize, for example, that their problem began not three months ago, or six months ago, but several years ago. Thus, at its best, the taking of the history is a two-way learning process: We as physicians learn about the more subtle aspects of our patient's problems, while the patients become more sensitized to their symptoms and patterns.

One other point should be made. As we said, most of the patients we see have been previously treated for depression. Many of these people have been involved with one or more forms of psychotherapy, or "talk therapy." As such they have been exposed to a considerable degree of explaining things psychologically, even physical symptoms. These patients can be very adept at anticipating our questions and thus may provide answers that are at best confusing and at worst outright misleading. It is sometimes necessary for us to be alert to this tendency and work around it, either by asking questions in new ways or by taking some surprising directions in our conversations.

PHYSICAL EXAMINATION

After we have taken the patient's history, we will refer the patient for a thorough physical examination to make sure that no organic illness is present. Although it seems obvious to do so, it's an unfortunate fact that some psychiatrists are so focused on the mental aspects of mental illness that they may fail to uncover the possible physical causes of their patients' complaints. Yet physical and psychiatric illnesses can be intricately intertwined. It takes time, patience, and perception to sort them out.

For example, such physical conditions as thyroid disorders, hypoglycemia (low blood sugar), or infectious mononucleosis share certain symptoms in common with SAD, such as sustained decreases in energy and increased consumption of carbohydrates. While there is no laboratory test specifically designed to indicate the existence of SAD in an individual, blood or urine tests will usually reveal (or rule out) one of the other, more easily recognizable conditions. More specific tests can be ordered that will reveal the presence of viral invaders, such as Epstein-Barr virus, the cause of most cases of mononucleosis.

In diagnosing depression we focus particular attention on the thyroid. As many as ten million Americans, mostly women, may suffer from a thyroid condition. Surprisingly, as many as ten to fifteen percent of patients who demonstrate symptoms of depression actually are suffering from a malfunctioning thyroid gland. This powerful gland, part of the endocrine system, is situated at the base of the neck, lying across the windpipe just below the larynx.

The thyroid's job is to secrete hormones called T3 and T4. These powerful chemicals regulate the activity of every cell in the body, including cells in the brain, and thus are essential for growth, development, and body metabolism. The chain of events that triggers thyroid secretion of hormones is as follows: In the brain the hypothalamus, cued by the various signals that monitor body function, releases thyrotropin-releasing hormone (TRH). TRH then travels to the neighboring pituitary gland, where it triggers the release of thyroid stimulating hormone (TSH). TSH then travels to the thyroid, which begins production of T3 and T4. In addition to regulating cell metabolism, these hormones also serve to "switch off" the pituitary when adequate bloodstream levels have been reached.

However, due to a number of causes, ranging from a genetic defect to a deficiency in the essential nutrient iodine, the thyroid can malfunction. When this happens, it either releases insufficient supplies of hormones (hypothyroidism) or it floods the body with them (hyperthyroidism). In either condition, the only symptoms that someone may notice are primarily psychiatric: depression or fatigue, or both. Other symptoms common to both hypothyroidism and depression include constipation, decreased libido, decreased concentration, and in some cases suicidal ideation and delusions.

Consequently when we encounter patients with symptoms of depression we automatically order a lab procedure known as the thyroid-releasing hormone (TRH) test to assess their thyroid function. This test first measures the level of thyroid stimulating hormone (TSH) currently present in the bloodstream. Then the patient is given an injection of synthetic TRH. Normally, after such an injection, TSH shows a rapid rise, peaking about thirty minutes later and returning to normal within about two hours. In people with hypothyroidism, however, the rise in TSH is much greater.

Hyperthyroidism, which has not been studied to as great an extent as hypothyroidism, can cause a person to feel anxious and irritable, and may induce frequent mood swings or emotional explosions. Sometimes the condition is misdiagnosed as mania or psychosis. Depression is another symptom that is frequently reported. In people with hyperthyroidism, the TRH test will result in only slight changes in the level of TSH. Paradoxically, in as many as one out of four depressed patients with normal thyroids, the TRH test will also produce only slight TSH changes. Such results are so consistent that they have come to be viewed as a "marker," a sign that biological depression is present.

There is another test that is often used in diagnosing biological depression: the dexamethasone suppression test, or DST. The DST is the subject of considerable controversy in the medical profession; it is generally considered to be helpful, however, in helping to recognize depression that is biological in origin, as opposed to depression that arises purely from mental or situational causes. Biologic depression is sometimes known as endogenous depression. (Endogenous means "arising from within," or, as the DSM-III-R labels it, depression of the melancholic type.)

Because they are caused by a chemical malfunction, endogenous depressions usually respond to medical treatments that restore chemical balance, such as the use of antidepressants. SAD is a form of endogenous depression that responds to light. Situational depressions usually respond to the use of psychotherapy, also known as "talk" therapy.

It has long been known that depressed people tend to secrete abnormally large amounts of cortisol due to overstimulation of hypothalamus, pituitary, and adrenal glands (the HPA axis). As we noted earlier, the feedback mechanism that tells the thermostat in the hypothalamus to shut off is faulty. (We should stress that the excess cortisol generated by this process does not directly produce symptoms of depression; it is merely a sign that the organs responsible for mood are out of kilter.) Dexamethasone is a potent corticosteroid that, when taken in pill form, affects the HPA axis and inhibits further production of the body's own cortisol. With the DST, the patient is given a small amount of dexamethasone at night. Over the next 24 hours the level of cortisol in the patient's blood is measured.

In people with depression, the HPA is different than in normal individuals—it is overactive, and thus produces large amounts of cortisol. This overproduction cannot be suppressed by administration of dexamethasone. Thus cortisol levels that are still abnormally high the next day are one clue that the patient does indeed suffer from some kind of mental illness. As a rule, the less cortisol suppression and the higher the cortisol levels, the more severe the illness.

Statistically the DST can only be relied on to detect about half of the cases of biological depression. The results of the DST and the TRH tests together, however, may identify as many as

85 percent of unipolar depressives. Adding confusion to the diagnostic picture is the fact, unearthed by some recent studies, that patients with SAD will generally (but not always) show *normal* results following the dexamethasone suppression test. In other words, in some SAD patients, as in healthy people, dexamethasone *does* suppress, or cause a reduction in, cortisol levels.

As we mentioned, the importance of the use of the DST in routine clinical practice is controversial, and results must be interpreted with caution. Researchers are beginning to find that cortisol levels can be affected by a number of factors, including hospitalization, age, and the severity of the patient's illness. People who have lost weight recently are also more likely to have abnormal DST results.

Also, like many other organic processes, the secretion of cortisol (and thus its suppression) is subject to control by circadian rhythms; some evidence even suggests cortisol levels fluctuate with the seasons over the course of a year. One controversial study reports having found that patients with a certain form of depression showed somewhat more normal results on their DST during the summer compared with winter.

One final note on this point: A recent study reported on a patient with SAD who, unlike most patients with the disorder, showed abnormal DST results. This same patient did not respond to the light therapy alone that had proved so helpful to so many others. While a single patient anecdote hardly constitutes scientific proof, further research may one day indicate whether DST results, or the findings of some other tests such as the TRH test, will help predict which patients are most likely to respond to light therapy and which may require additional treatments.

To summarize: The dexamethasone suppression test can be used as part of the effort to detect the presence of endogenous depression in roughly 50 percent of patients. A positive result on the test usually occurs in cases where the depression has become particularly severe. The depression seen in SAD, while very troubling to those it afflicts, is rated as less severe than other types of major depression. Moreover, patients with SAD will usually not demonstrate positive findings on a DST. If, on the other hand, positive results do occur, we need to consider whether a patient's SAD symptoms are merely the outward presentation of a deeper form of illness.

Depending on such findings—and spurred by our suspicions—we refer patients for other types of tests in order to discover whether their depression has some physical cause. For example, the radiological technique known as a computerized transverse axial tomography (usually blessedly shortened to CAT or CT scan) enables us to take detailed pictures of tissues, including the brain, without the use of contrast dyes. A CAT scan can detect tumors, hemorrhages, blood vessel blockage, or areas where blood may have collected due to injury. Any of these conditions can cause at least some of the symptoms associated with depression.

Similarly, we will usually order an electroencephalograph (EEG) so as to rule out the presence of a seizure disorder. During an EEG, electrodes placed on different parts of the skull detect and record electric signals generated by brain activity. Any signs of abnormal activity may indicate that the patient suffers from epilepsy, tumor, infection, or hemorrhage. In some cases knowing the exact site of any unusual activity—technically known as the seizure focus—can help us identify the presence of a specific ailment. For example, the EEG can pinpoint the site of temporal lobe epilepsy (TLE), a seizure disorder that involves an area on the side of the brain and produces a distinctive pattern of symptoms, some of which include mood instability and depression.

PSYCHIATRIC EVALUATION

In some cases, after we have taken the history, referred the patient for a physical examination, and ruled out the presence of organic disease, we may decide it would be useful to conduct one or more psychiatric evaluations to determine the nature and scope of the depression. Until recently, one such tool used by psychiatrists was the Hamilton Rating Scale, a standardized questionnaire designed to evaluate a person's mood. The higher the score on this test, the more severe the illness. By repeating this rating assessment over the course of time, psychiatrists got a picture of how a patient's depression was affecting him or her on a particular day and thus evaluated the impact of changing conditions, including the time of year.

However, as we have seen, SAD is characterized by a number of features that place it in a different category than other forms of depression. And the Hamilton Scale has not been revised recently to accommodate the updated definitions of depression as contained in the DSM-III-R. It is therefore less sensitive to the pattern of symptoms found in SAD and thus may not generate positive findings, despite a patient's profound symptomatology. Consequently the Hamilton Scale or other similar assessment devices by themselves will not paint a complete picture of the SAD patient.

To compensate for this problem, SAD experts have designed several supplementary rating scales. One such tool, developed by Dr. Frederick M. Jacobsen and Dr. Norman Rosenthal, lists seven items usually associated with SAD but not with most other forms of depression. Patients are interviewed in the following areas:

- Fatigue, low energy level, feelings of heaviness in the limbs, being laden, "weighed down." Such feelings are rated on a scale ranging from "Does not feel more fatigued than usual" to "Fatigued almost all the time."
- Social withdrawal (ranging from "Interacts with other people as usual" to "Marked withdrawal from others in family or work situations")
- Appetite increase (from "No increase in appetite" to "Wants to eat much more than usual")
- Increased eating (from "Is not eating more than usual" to "Is eating much more than usual")

- Carbohydrate craving (from "No change in food preference" to "Irresistible craving for sweets or starches")
- Weight gain (from "No weight gain" to "Definite weight gain")
- Hypersomnia (from "No increase in sleep length" to "Four or more hours increase in sleep length")

Another tool some psychiatrists use, one developed by Drs. Rosenthal, Gary Bradt, and Thomas Wehr, is known as the Seasonal Pattern Assessment Questionnaire (SPAQ); it is designed to reveal how a patient's depression changes over the course of the year.

Among the questions covered by SPAQ:

- How many years have you lived in this climatic area?
- To what degree do the following change with the seasons (rated from "No Change" to "Extremely Marked Change"): Sleep length, social activity, mood, weight, appetite, energy level.
- In which month do you:
  Feel best
  Tend to gain most weight
  Socialize most
  Sleep least
  Eat most
  Lose most weight
  Socialize least
  Feel worst
  Eat least
  Sleep most
- Indicate how weather changes make you feel (rated from "In very low spirits or markedly slowed down" to "markedly improves mood or energy level"):
  Cold weather
  Hot weather
  Humid weather
  Sunny days

Dry days
Gray, cloudy days
Long days
High pollen count
Foggy, smoggy days
Short days

- By how much does your weight fluctuate during the course of the year?
- Including naps, how many hours a day do you sleep during each season?
- Do you notice a change in food preference during the different seasons? What are the specific changes?
- If you experience changes with the seasons, do you feel that these are a problem for you? If yes, how severe (from mild to disabling)?

DIFFERENTIAL DIAGNOSIS: DISTINGUISHING SAD FROM OTHER RELATED ILLNESSES

Depending on the information gathered during the preceding steps, we will begin to be able to differentiate whether they are truly afflicted by SAD, or whether some other more subtle variety of depression is present. We should take a moment to describe some of these other conditions.

The craving for carbohydrates, for example, might indicate that some form of eating disorder is present. Other clues to such a disorder would include obesity or excessive thinness, remarks (most often made by women) that the patient perceives herself as "fat" when she is obviously not, a preoccupation with body size or excessive concern about physical appearance, or a pattern of binge eating. One tipoff to a certain type of eating disorder, one in which the patient is extremely concerned about weight, is that the patient exercises excessively. In fact, to these people, exercise is at least as important to them as not eating.

Obviously, such a symptom would help differentiate between an eating disorder and SAD, in which most patients can barely drag themselves into work, let alone exercise for two or three hours a day.

As we have stated, sleep disturbances are a feature in many types of depression. In SAD disturbed sleep takes a specific form, that of daytime sleepiness (hypersomnia) or difficulty rising in the morning. But such hypersomnia might be the result of other conditions. Many people snore, but some snoring is caused by blocked breathing passages and results in a condition known as sleep apnea. People with this disorder wake themselves up hundreds of times during the course of a single night in order to get enough oxygen to stay alive. During these frequent wakenings patients don't quite reach consciousness; their sleep pattern is disturbed and they awaken feeling unrefreshed, a feeling that persists throughout the day.

There is an entire spectrum of other sleep disturbances that have other causes and require other cures. Insomnia, for example, might take the form of difficulty falling asleep at night, or difficulty staying asleep once sleep is achieved. It might also mean waking in the early hours of the morning and not being able to return to sleep. And a small percentage of insomniacs suffer from disturbed circadian rhythms; their metabolic processes simply can't work in harmony to produce sleep at the appropriate times. Each of these conditions requires a different diagnostic procedure and a therapeutic strategy. Snoring, for example, may need surgical correction, while insomnia usually responds to a change in daytime or nighttime habits, psychiatric counseling, or, in some cases, medication.

As our understanding of SAD grows, so does our awareness that it, like other illnesses, can affect people with differing degrees of severity. The spectrum of SAD-like disorders, in other words, may represent a range from mild to virtually debilitating. While some researchers have not yet been convinced that SAD really exists as a clinically definable subtype of depression, others have identified what they believe are distinct variations on the illness. If these variations exist, then they, too, will need to be differentiated so that proper treatment can be prescribed.

For example, in some quarters, "winter blues" is given the somewhat more technical, if less colorful, name "sub-syndromal SAD" or S-SAD. As its name implies, S-SAD is less intense and less crippling than SAD. Patients with S-SAD do not experience the same difficulty in functioning or concentrating as those with a full-blown case of the disorder. They do, however, become less energetic, less efficient, and less sociable as winter marches on; they may even experience increased appetite and increased sleepiness. And also like their SAD-afflicted cousins, they appear to respond to light therapy. In another part of this book we mentioned cabin fever—those feelings of boredom, edginess and stress resulting from isolation, lack of mental and physical exercise. It appears that some investigators feel that cabin fever represents a kind of "sub-sub-syndromal SAD."

Interestingly, Dr. Thomas Wehr has identified a syndrome that he calls "reverse SAD." In this disorder, patients experience the same symptoms as SAD but at completely opposite times of the year: Their depressions appear in the summer and remit during the fall and winter. People with reverse SAD actually get worse under the standard regimen of phototherapy used to treat "normal" SAD. Because of their sensitivity to light, these patients tend to wear tinted lenses, and often wear sunglasses even while indoors. As an experiment, Dr. Wehr asked one reverse-SAD patient, then suffering from an episode of summer depression, to stay indoors in an air-conditioned apartment, periodically exposing herself to very cold temperatures. After five days the patient's mood improved considerably, only to relapse nine days after treatment was discontinued.

Dr. Alfred Lewy, who discovered that light suppresses melatonin secretion, has proposed that SAD patients be further categorized according to the apparent disruption in their circadian rhythms: whether they are "phase-advanced" (that is, their rhythms peak earlier than normal) or "phase-delayed" (their rhythms peak later than normal). This information, he argues, can be important in selecting the time of day at which therapy, particularly light therapy, may be most beneficial.

We would like to mention one final SAD variation, one that was first described by two of our colleagues in New Jersey, Dr. Peter Mueller and N. Grace Allen. Some time before SAD emerged as a recognized form of depression, they reported on a patient suffering from a condition they called Seasonal Energy Syndrome (SES). The patient experienced fall-winter symptoms of energy loss, depressed mood, hypersomnia, cravings for sugar, weight gain, and impaired concentration; in the spring, the patient experienced insomnia, elevated mood, absence of sugar cravings, and weight loss. Fall/winter symptoms grew more severe the further north the patient lived. Sound familiar? The patient's condition was relieved through the use of phototherapy. It seems clear that the seasonal energy syndrome they had identified in this patient, which was subsequently detected in other people by other researchers, was virtually identical to the disorder that was soon to become more widely known as SAD.

In a subsequent study of 47 patients, however, Mueller and Allen identified an even more serious form of SES. Patients with this disorder tend to have a high incidence of psychosis, violent actions, suicide attempts, temporal lobe epilepsy (TLE), migraine, chemical addiction, attention deficits, and a history of multiple and/or long-term hospitalizations in psychiatric institutes. In the fall and winter, people with SES often manifest signs of a condition called Raynaud's phenomenon, a disorder of the circulation that can result in paleness or blueness in the fingers and toes during exposure to cold or during emotional upset. They are also more easily bruised during this time of year compared to the summer months. During the spring and summer, SES patients exhibit such symptoms as hyperactivity, insomnia, high sex drive, weight loss, anorexia, migraine, elevated moods, and episodes of violence.

Identifying these distinct types of seasonal disorders is not just an exercise in psychiatric hairsplitting: quite the contrary. As it turns out, patients with severe SES do not respond to the full-spectrum light therapy used in the treatment of SAD. In fact, the use of such lights can be counterproductive, tending to exacerbate their symptoms rather than relieve them.

Mueller and Allen found instead that patients with SES benefit from an innovative and somewhat surprising treatment approach. During the fall and winter, they had their patients wear glasses containing rose-colored lenses, which filtered sunlight so that only the red parts of the spectrum penetrated the eye. Use of these glasses alleviated most of the symptoms. Conversely the use of glasses with blue-green lenses during the spring and summer lessened the severity of the symptoms associated with that time of year. This manipulation of natural light was supplemented with the use of antiseizure medications and other chemicals, including tryptophan.

As you certainly realize by now, pinning down the diagnosis of SAD can be a knotty problem. Once the diagnosis has been confirmed, however, treatment can be prescribed. Before therapy begins, however, there is one more step to be taken.

TELLING THE PATIENT

At this point in the process, having conducted our examination and considered the possibilities, we have sufficient information to make the diagnosis of Seasonal Affective Disorder. We must then share our finding with the patient. Some of our patients have heard of SAD, through articles in the newspaper or reports on television or through previous involvement in the psychotherapeutic process. Others have not.

We give our patients as much information as we can about their condition, giving careful answers to their questions and explaining how their symptoms are caused by a biological malfunctioning, not a defect in their personality. To those who are interested, we distribute copies of articles explaining the origin, symptoms, and treatment of the disorder. Many patients read such articles and recognize themselves in the descriptions of SAD patients.

In almost every case, the reaction to our diagnosis is one of relief. Many times we have heard patients say that they had begun to give up hope, that they had tried everything they could to relieve their depression and felt they would never really feel like themselves again. Characteristically patients express joy in hearing that they are not alone, that other people who have suffered from the same condition have been helped and have gotten better.

For these patients, the treatment we prescribe is, literally, the light at the end of the tunnel, as explained in the next chapter.

Chapter 6

SHEDDING LIGHT ON SAD

Like many other psychiatrists, we admit we were somewhat surprised when we first heard about the dramatic improvements experienced by patients with Seasonal Affective Disorder who were treated with one of nature's oldest and simplest remedies: light. Yet as clinicians we are concerned with helping our patients. If a technique stands a chance of succeeding, we are willing to give it a try, especially in cases where the patient has not improved as much as would be hoped under other types of treatment.

Our results, as well as those from other physicians around the world, have strongly confirmed the validity of the phototherapeutic approach. As physicians we take a certain pride in being able to improve the outlook for patients with this disorder using a "medicine" that is highly effective, fast-acting, relatively inexpensive, and virtually free of troubling side effects.

At Fair Oaks, almost all of our seriously depressed patients require medication; these may include antidepressants, antiseizure medications, or lithium. In addition, depending on the situation, they participate in several forms of talk therapy. Yet as we have noted, most of the patients for whom SAD is a significant factor never get 100 percent better through the use of these conventional strategies. Only when phototherapy is added to the regimen do these patients experience the desired improvement in mood. Such results, replicated in other centers here and abroad, are convincing proof that light is a tremendously effective treatment and a powerful tool for managing this particular illness.

Further evidence of phototherapy's benefits comes from the remarks made by patients. One patient described a flood of energy felt within days of therapy. "You can't imagine the relief," she said, while a second patient said that use of the lights "is like a gift someone has given me. I get back four months a year that I never had."

In addition to its efficacy, light therapy has a number of other positive aspects that recommend it as the ideal treatment strategy for SAD. Patients notice improvement very quickly—sometimes after the first session, and usually within two to four days. Medications, in contrast, require between ten days and four weeks to take effect. Significantly, patients don't develop a tolerance to light; in other words, they don't need to constantly increase the dose as time goes on, although they do require more light in direct relationship to the severity of their depression. Apart from the initial medical evaluation, the purchase of equipment and medical monitoring, continued light therapy is relatively inexpensive.

What's more, patients can conduct the therapy in their own homes; they are usually able to develop a personal treatment strategy that fits their normal schedules and activities. Many patients thus come to feel that phototherapy is a form of treatment over which they have some control. Administering light is something they can do for themselves.

Despite its elegant simplicity, however, phototherapy is not just a matter of turning on a lamp and basking in the glow. It is a recognized therapeutic technique that must be administered by a trained medical professional. Considerable research has been conducted in the past decade to study the type of light required, the method of delivery, and the dosage—intensity, timing, and duration of exposure. Notwithstanding these efforts, many questions remain unanswered, and a great deal of controversy still exists among experts concerning the exact strategy that produces the greatest benefit. In this chapter we will outline the phototherapy regimen we use and discuss variations in the approaches used by other researchers in the field. In a subsequent chapter we will discuss the other vital components of SAD therapy, including the use of medication and psychiatric counseling.

COVERING THE SPECTRUM

As we have seen, SAD is considered to be a disruption in the circadian rhythms, particularly those that govern the brain chemistry responsible for our mood. Research on circadian rhythms has shown that circadian entrainment—the process by which we "set" our biological clocks—occurs as a response to light.

Experiments demonstrate that the effects of light on this entraining process, and thus its antidepressant effects, are transmitted through the eyes and not by the skin. In one such experiment, subjects wearing swimsuits were exposed to light for several hours a day over a seven-day period. While the face, neck, arms, and legs were exposed, their eyes were shielded with goggles that admitted only enough light to permit the subjects to watch television. Then, for another week, the situation was reversed: their eyes were unshielded, while the rest of the face and body was completely covered. Of the nine people tested, seven experienced a response to the "eye treatment" only; one responded to the "skin treatment," while another one responded to both approaches.

The eyes are exquisitely sensitive to the spectrum of light emanating from a given source. Experiments have shown that even small changes in spectral composition can affect both the emotional and physical responses of the body to light. If you remember from the discussion in Chapter 5, patients with Seasonal Energy Syndrome improve dramatically while wearing glasses with rose-colored lenses in the fall and winter, and with blue-green lenses in the spring and summer.

Phototherapy is intended to replicate the so-called "white" light generated naturally by the sun. Thus the bulbs used are known as "full-spectrum" bulbs because the light they produce contains a more natural range of light (including some ultraviolet, or UV) than normal indoor lighting. While experts are not yet certain exactly which part of the spectrum produces the therapeutic response, some evidence suggests that the red wavelengths are involved. Studies are also under way to determine whether the UV component plays any role in producing the antidepressant response.

There are two main types of bulbs used for illumination: incandescent and fluorescent. The bulbs used in phototherapy are fluorescent tubes.

Incandescents—the pear-shaped bulbs found in most lamps—contain a twisted filament, usually made of tungsten, that glows as current passes through it. As you know if you've ever tried to change a bulb that has just been burning, these bulbs generate a great deal of heat. The laws of physics dictate that radiation produced by such hot sources occurs primarily on the red end of the spectrum. In fact, about 90 percent of the radiation emitted from an incandescent bulb falls in the infrared (beyond visible red) spectrum. Incandescent light thus contains more yellow and less blue than sunlight.

Fluorescents work on a completely different principle. Rather than containing a filament, a fluorescent tube is filled with gas, such as argon or neon. The surface of the tube is coated with a substance known as a phosphor. Electricity passing through the tube strips electrons from the molecules of gas. These electrons then go flying through the phosphorous coating, exciting it and causing it to emit light. The wavelength of the light depends on the exact composition of the phosphor. A television screen, for example, contains three different phosphors—one for red, one for green, and one for blue. One primary advantage of fluorescents is that they produce virtually no heat.

As we mentioned, the tubes used in phototherapy are specially designed to emit white light that roughly approximates sunlight and are different from the tubes typically used in homes and offices. Those lights are called "cool white" because they emit light concentrated in the blue part of the spectrum, eliminating much of the red and yellow wavelengths and all of the UV radiation. Lighting engineers use sunlight as a standard for measuring the color range of a light source; the sun thus is said to have a "color index" of 100. The bulbs used in phototherapy (specifically the brand known as "Vita-Lites") have a color index of 91; the next closest variety has a color index of only 68. Also, phototherapy bulbs are known in the industry as "powertwist" tubes because they are twisted in such a way as to increase the surface area covered by phosphors, and thus emit even more light.

The intensity of light is measured in units called "lux." Typical indoor lighting in the home or office usually registers at between 100 (the minimum needed for reading) and 500 lux. Compare these low levels to the 10,000 lux or more you would see while standing outside on a cloudless day. Even standing at a window on a sunny day, you are exposed to light of 2500 lux. The Vita-Lites used in phototherapy generate light of 2500 lux intensity measured at a distance of three feet.

DESIGNING THE PHOTOTHERAPY REGIMEN

Typically the course of light therapy at Fair Oaks follows this pattern:

First, of course, we assemble all the evidence we can about the patient's condition, including the history and the results of the physical examination. Having confirmed the diagnosis of SAD, we schedule a session with the patient to discuss the condition and its treatment. One of us (Dr. McGuire) keeps a set of lights in her office. At the beginning of the session she will explain the concepts involved and ask the patient's permission to switch on the lights. We might tell the patient, for example, that his or her response to previous therapy demonstrates a pattern much like that of other patients with SAD, and that light therapy has a chance of producing some benefits.

Not surprisingly, many patients consider phototherapy to be a rather eccentric or peculiar notion—to put it mildly. Of course, for the most part, these are people who over the years have seen a number of physicians, have tried numerous medications, and have engaged in round after round of psychotherapy. To them, such a radically different approach to treatment can seem futile at best. Our patients' responses to the notion of phototherapy have ranged from mild amusement to outright disbelief. Some may even consider the technique to be a form of "black magic." Nonetheless, we use our best efforts to convince them of the merits of phototherapy. Once this hurdle has been surmounted, the lights are switched on and the session continues.

During this time we keep alert to any changes in the patient's personality. It is at this point that our skills as clinical observers are most acutely challenged. Sometimes, for example, a change might occur in the pace at which the patient speaks, or the way he or she sits in the chair. At other times we detect a slightly different expression in the patient's face or eyes: There may be more color in the face, or the patient looks less tired. In some cases a clue may be found in the way a patient uses a certain characteristic hand gestures. In any event, such changes may be barely perceptible—but they are there.

Not infrequently, at the end of the session, patients comment that they feel much better. But they usually deny that the lights had anything to do with it; instead they attribute improvement to talk therapy. However, if we have noted any changes, regardless of how subtle, we suggest that the patient return over the next five to seven days for a more formalized course of phototherapy.

These subsequent sessions take place in a room at Fair Oaks that has been adapted to the use of the lights. As a rule the goal is to make phototherapy as convenient for the patient as possible; thus with some patients we schedule sessions to coincide with the lunch hour.

The patient sits in front of a "light box," a metal frame measuring 2.5 by 4 feet. The box contains eight Vita-Lite tubes covered by a plastic diffuser that distributes the light evenly across the surface. Behind the tubes is a surface designed to reflect as much light as possible through the diffusing screen. Recently an improved light unit has become available that measures 1.5 by 4 feet and weighs less than the original model. Such refinements in equipment continue to make light therapy easier and more convenient for patients, especially for home use.

A phototherapy session usually lasts an hour. During this time the patients sits about 3 feet away from the light unit and is allowed to read, knit, work a puzzle, or talk on the telephone. Any activity is all right, so long as patients don't sleep or close their eyes. The only other requirement is that they sit facing the lights and glance at the screen for ten or fifteen seconds out of every minute. It is not necessary, and may actually be harmful, to stare at the light constantly.

Usually we notice significant improvement in the patient by the third or fourth day. Of course such improvement depends on a number of factors, including the severity of the patient's depression, the regimen of prescribed medications, problems at home, and so on. The actual degree of improvement is not really the issue, however. What we are looking for, as we would with any medication is a *trend* toward improvement.

During this week we monitor the patient's response to therapy closely in order to adjust the dosage to the proper level. If a patient remarks, for example, that he or she used the lights for an hour the day before and still felt depressed, then we suggest the sessions be extended to ninety minutes or two hours. Such fine-tuning continues until patients reach the mood they consider normal for themselves.

One way of recognizing that dosage is too high is to watch for signs of overstimulation: rapid speech, quick movements. Often the patients themselves are not aware that they are being overstimulated, and must be taught to recognize the signs. We then work together to adjust the period of light exposure.

Despite our best efforts, not all patients in whom we might have predicted a response to phototherapy show a trend toward improvement. Most do, however. If over the course of the week we spot that trend, we encourage those of our patients who are about to be discharged to invest in a set of lights for use at home. The cost, around four hundred dollars, is minimal compared to the benefits gained.

During this phase of treatment—known as the maintenance phase—we work closely with patients to design a course of phototherapy that can be integrated as easily as possible into their lifestyles. For example, we don't necessarily insist that exposure to the lights occur during a particular time of day, although for those people who work it certainly makes sense to use the lights before leaving the house in the morning. As we tell them, why drag yourself through your day at work when the lights can help prepare you for the stresses that await you on the job? Similarly, we urge patients to avoid use of the lights too late at night, since overstimulation may make it difficult to fall asleep. And of course, poor sleep one night leads to excessive sleepiness the following day.

Fortunately most of our patients' families are more than willing to make the few small adjustments needed in their own lives and schedules to help their depressed relative take advantage of phototherapy. For example, a father might agree to prepare breakfast and get the kids ready for school so that the mother can have an uninterrupted session in front of the lights. Most people find that bright lights don't bother them, especially when they realize the improvement they bring about in the depressed relative.

Over the course of the winter we continue to monitor their use of and response to phototherapy. One mechanism for doing so is usually already in place, since we continue to meet for weekly psychotherapy sessions during which we discuss progress. However we also make ourselves available to our patients by phone. We frequently receive calls, for example, during which the patient reports feeling overstimulated, or remarks that the effect seems to be wearing off. We will then offer advice on ways to improve the effectiveness of the treatment.

Our patients are told to continue using the lights throughout the dark months until they begin to feel they no longer need them. For some people this moment might occur as early as February; for others it might not take place until the end of April. One way we recognize that the moment to terminate phototherapy has arrived is if the patient reports feeling overstimulated after a session. Should that occur we will suggest tapering back on the amount of exposure time, or stopping the therapy altogether.

Once the symptoms abate, most patients remain free of depression as long as they continue to use the lights. However, one problem we frequently face, not just with phototherapy but with all antidepressant regimens, is patient compliance: the willingness to go along with the physician's plan for treatment. Should patients terminate therapy before the end of winter for any reason—travel, family obligations, or just plain forgetfulness—they will usually relapse within three days. Sometimes patients simply misunderstand the instructions they have been given about how to use the lights. Renewed use of lights will again begin to alleviate depression; often, though, it can take up to three days for the full effects of phototherapy to return.

Another problem of compliance, one peculiar to depression, should be mentioned at this point. People who suffer from mood swings tend to forget, during their low periods, what it was like when they felt "normal." In the depths of depression they can no longer remember that they ever felt happy, or that certain treatments worked for them. A sense of helplessness, hopelessness, and despair can permeate every facet of their existence. Consequently they might forget, for example, that phototherapy ever helped to alleviate their depression and thus begin to neglect their treatment. Should that happen we begin the process all over again: We must demonstrate to the patient that phototherapy alleviates depression, reschedule sessions with the lights, and work again to achieve the proper elevation of mood. The process can be frustrating but the rewards are well worth the effort.

The approach to phototherapy we've just outlined is the one we have found most effective for our patients. We should stress again, however, that each patient has different needs that must be taken into account. For example, some people have jobs whose schedules make it difficult to sit before the lights at prescribed times. Others find it hard to undergo therapy at home and still manage to cope with the demands of their families. We work closely with our patients to establish the most effective strategy, one that recognizes the realities of their lives without losing sight of the important goal of relieving depression.

In addition to phototherapy, there are many other steps that can be taken to alleviate the symptoms of SAD. Foremost, of course, is that the patient continues to follow the regimen of antidepressant medications we have prescribed, and that participation continue in any recommended course of psychotherapy. We'll expand on this in Chapter 7. But there are many commonsense strategies as well. We urge our patients to get outside as much as possible during the winter months, especially in the morning. For a few people a walk at sunrise may be enough to relieve feelings of depression. For others, of course, especially those for whom hypersomnia is a problem, the thought of rising so early can pose a problem. As we indicated earlier, however, regular bedtimes and strict limits on the number of hours of sleep can actually help alleviate daytime sleepiness.

And some patients enjoy participation in winter sports—skiing, hiking, and so on. The added exposure to sunlight (especially if it is being reflected off of snow) is helpful, and there are the added benefits of exercise, a change in routine, social contact, and of course the fun that sports provide. We also urge that patients rearrange the furniture in their homes and offices so that they face windows as much as possible. While it should not need mentioning, we always caution patients never to glance directly at the sun for any reason.

At this point we should remind you that depressive episodes in SAD are triggered not by winter per se but by the reduced amount of sunlight available during the shortened days of the cold season. Because this is true, a person with SAD can be affected even during the dog days of August, should a period of cloudy weather persist for more than a few days. Patients who have purchased a set of phototherapy lights for use in the home may thus want to use them to ward off the depressive effects of an extended period of reduced sunlight.

Some people have installed fluorescent light fixtures with full-spectrum bulbs for use in their homes or places of work. However *we strongly advise against doing so*. There are too many factors, such as timing and intensity of exposure, that are not under control. Without adequate supervision, phototherapy poses the risk of overstimulation. The uncontrolled use of such fixtures throughout the home is certainly no substitute for a medically correct regimen of phototherapy undertaken in consultation with a doctor.

QUESTIONS AND CONTROVERSIES

At this point we should note that the science of photomedicine is a very recent development. As in any new field of medicine, experts are not in complete agreement concerning the therapeutic strategy that will produce the most benefit for the greatest number of SAD patients. Even as this book is being written, studies are under way at a number of research centers to resolve some of these controversies and determine the optimal phototherapy regimen. Among the questions still to be resolved: At what time of day is exposure to light likely to be most effective? How bright should the lights be? How long should a patient be exposed? Is full-spectrum light necessary, or should ultraviolet radiation be eliminated? What are the long-term risks of phototherapy? What medications or other therapeutic strategies might supplement the use of lights? A brief discussion of these questions will help shed some light, if we may use that phrase, on the nature of SAD and the evolving theories of its treatment.

Consider, for instance, the matter of timing. Is phototherapy more effective in the morning or evening? Does light have therapeutic value because it resets our biological clocks, or simply because it extends the "photoperiod"—that portion of the day during which we are exposed to light? Or is light beneficial regardless of the time of exposure? And what about such factors as the quantity of light, measured in length of exposure, or the quality, as measured by intensity and the spectrum generated by the bulbs?

The answers are significant for several reasons. As we have seen, one effect of light is to entrain our circadian rhythms. It may be that our internal clocks will react to light at certain times (in the morning, say) and not at others. Thus light given in the morning may work, while light at other times may not.

This may be especially true if disturbances in the cycle of melatonin secretion ultimately prove to be the cause of SAD. As we discussed earlier, melatonin secretion in healthy people begins with the onset of darkness, whereas in most people with SAD secretion begins much later in the night. Studies show that morning light exposure advances the time at which melatonin is secreted (in other words, it moves the start of secretion back a few hours) but that evening light delays it. Since melatonin plays a role in regulating moods, "normalizing" this rhythm may be a factor in alleviating depression. Other researchers disagree, however, citing studies that show light administered during the afternoon, when no melatonin is being secreted, can still produce an antidepressant effect.

Another reason the question of timing and duration is important is that some patients would deem it a hardship to rise every morning at five or six o'clock—before sunup—to sit in front of lights for several hours. Many people would no doubt find it easier to comply with a regimen of afternoon light therapy, providing it was just as effective and would not interfere with work.

Some experts find that timing is not a critical issue, that light relieves SAD regardless of the time of day it is given. We at Fair Oaks tend to support this view. Others, however, believe that morning therapy is better. They cite evidence showing that most SAD patients have delayed circadian rhythms, which need to be shifted so as to operate on an earlier cycle. Some hold that evening light alone may do the trick, and may improve patient compliance, but that the use of light during both the morning and evening light is best.

Research on the matter of timing has produced conflicting evidence, which only serves to fuel the controversy. In one study, for example, a patient exposed to four hours of light in the morning and another four in the evening experienced complete remission of symptoms. Two more patients in the study, however, reported feeling overstimulated and had trouble sleeping after five hours of light a day; these problems abated when they cut back to just three hours in the evening only. Other researchers found that the antidepressant response to evening and morning light therapy is better than just evening alone. One team of investigators found evidence that light given in the early afternoon produced just as much therapeutic benefits as morning light, and that it did so without causing any shift in circadian rhythms. They concluded that it may not be necessary to extend the light exposure through morning and evening exposure to lights.

Perhaps the only solid conclusion that can be drawn from such conflicting findings is that each patient will respond to treatment in a different way; care must therefore be taken to tailor the regimen to suit the individual. Our approach is to give phototherapy at a time that is most convenient for the patient. If it works, fine; we carry on. If no effect is noticed, then the patient can be shifted to therapy at another time of day.

Let's discuss the matter of intensity. As we stated earlier, the usual approach is to use bright lights rated at 2500 lux at a distance of three feet. Most studies confirm that dim light (100-300 lux) is ineffective in alleviating depression. However, a report from Switzerland indicates that some SAD patients responded to the use of dim yellow light. It is possible that such unusual findings were the result of other variables besides the brightness of the lights. Specifically, this group of patients may have been less severely ill than those in other studies, or they may have been sitting closer to the light source. Even the size of the patients' pupils may have affected the amount of light they received.

A physician in the New York area is currently treating his SAD patients using light of very high intensity: 10,000 lux, equivalent to the light you would see if you stood in shade on a sunny day, and four times as bright as that used in most other treatment centers. He reports that his patients appear to improve with just thirty minutes of exposure a day. Whether such intensive therapy is free of long-term risk, such as retinal damage, has not yet been demonstrated.

One other aspect that must be considered about light intensity is the fact that some depressed patients, particularly those with a bipolar disorder such as manic-depressive illnesses, are hypersensitive to light. Some of these patients are known to become hypomanic during the summer months. It is therefore conceivable that some SAD patients are also extremely sensitive to light. Normal therapeutic doses may be too stimulating for these people, who may be helped by light at considerably lower intensities.

As you have seen, the duration of exposure is also a subject of debate. There are reports of patients benefiting from as little as thirty minutes or an hour to as much as eight hours of phototherapy a day. It appears, however, that most people benefit from between one and two hours of light exposure a day; for some the amount is between two and five hours. Some researchers hold that longer durations seem to be more effective than shorter ones. The duration of exposure needed to produce an antidepressant response is no doubt a factor of the light's intensity; a half-hour of 10,000 lux light may one day prove to be just as effective as two hours of light at 2500 lux.

There are other factors to consider as well. One study found that patients' responses to phototherapy were directly related to the type of sleep disturbance they experienced as a result of SAD. For example, one patient who suffered from early morning insomnia (awakening too early and being unable to return to sleep) failed to respond to morning phototherapy but did respond to evening therapy. Conversely, a patient who tended to wake in the middle of the night showed no response to evening therapy but did benefit from morning therapy. One conclusion from such findings is that SAD patients may need to be classified according to the nature of their sleep disturbance in order to determine which phototherapy regimen is most likely to prove helpful.

While we're on the subject of sleep, we should point out that patients who rise early to undergo phototherapy obviously lose out on a certain amount of rest. And as we mentioned elsewhere in this book, one therapeutic strategy in managing depression is sleep deprivation. Researchers have determined, however, that the benefits of light therapy are not a direct result of sleep deprivation. For example, evening treatment produces benefits even though it usually causes patients to lose no sleep, nor is their sleep interrupted (except in cases of overstimulation).

As we explained earlier, we ask our patients to glance at the light source for ten to fifteen seconds out of every minute. To be honest, however, we don't actually know if looking directly at the light is necessary. It is not yet certain exactly how light needs to enter the eye, and where it needs to strike, in order to produce its therapeutic effect. It may indeed be true that light must follow a direct path between the source and the sensitive center of the retina, in which case glancing at the screen is necessary. However, we may yet determine that only the light receptors on the *periphery* of the retina may be involved, in which case light perceived through peripheral vision may be sufficient. If such is true, then looking directly at the lights would be unnecessary. Research to answer this question is currently under way.

A patient's age may also affect the therapeutic response. Some evidence suggests that children with SAD respond to phototherapy of shorter duration and of less intensity than adult patients. In fact, some children appear to do better with dim yellow light than with bright full-spectrum light, which in some young patients may prove to be overstimulating and interfere with sleep. We feel there is reason for concern that children of SAD patients who are exposed to phototherapy lights in the home may experience some degree of overstimulation. On the other end of the scale, the older the patient the more likely it is that he or she suffers from cataracts. The presence of cataracts will reduce the amount of light entering the eye and thus affect the patient's response to phototherapy.

As we have stated is the case in patients with Seasonal Energy Syndrome, light of different wavelengths may affect some people differently at different times of the year. Such patients notice relief from symptoms that occur in the fall (energy loss, hypersomnia, sugar cravings, and so on) when wearing rose-tinted lenses, which enhance the antidepressant effects of full-spectrum light. Conversely the symptoms that occur during spring (insomnia, weight loss, excessive elevation in mood) remit when patients wear glasses with blue-green lenses that filter out all red wavelengths.

As you can see, a great deal of controversy exists concerning virtually every aspect of phototherapy in the management of SAD, from the amount of light needed to the time of day it should be administered. Neither is it certain just how light works as an antidepressant, whether by correcting imbalances in circadian rhythms, or by artificially extending the illuminated portion of the day, or through some other means.

One fact, however, remains clear: phototherapy works. Since SAD was first recognized, physicians have used lights to treat hundreds of seasonally depressed patients. The overall efficacy rate is well over 80 percent, and in some studies approaches 100 percent.

Such results eliminate the possibility that most patients' responses to light are merely the result of a placebo effect—the power of suggestion. Scientists usually believe that a placebo response is likely to be present if a patient shows an immediate response to therapy. As a rule, however, while some effects can be noticed right away, phototherapy usually requires three or four days before it really begins to take hold. Dr. Norman Rosenthal has noted other characteristics that make a placebo effect unlikely. A placebo response usually occurs during the first course of therapy but not the second; with phototherapy, however, the response is constant from one course to the next, from one year to the next. In addition, relapse after withdrawal from treatment is considered to be a sign that the therapeutic benefit was real, not imaginary. As we mentioned, patients who stop using the lights almost always relapse within three days. Furthermore, placebo treatments usually will not prevent a disease from appearing; phototherapy however, is effective when used prophylactically to prevent the onset of symptoms.

Scientifically controlled studies have also shown that patient expectations do not play a role in determining the success of light treatment. In such studies patients are interviewed before therapy begins to determine what they expect might happen. For example, they might be told that they will be exposed to both yellow light and white light. They are then asked to predict which treatment they think will be more effective. Generally, their predictions fail to correspond with the actual outcome—in other words, those who guess that yellow light will work actually improve under white light. Again, such findings support the idea that phototherapy is genuinely effective, and not merely the result of the placebo effect.

SIDE EFFECTS AND OTHER CONCERNS

As with any therapy, however, there are some drawbacks associated with the use of lights. While the incidence of side effects is small, especially compared with the use of antidepressants or other medications, there are some hazards patients and physicians alike must be aware of when embarking on a regimen of phototherapy.

During the first or second day of therapy, for example, some patients may notice mild headaches that are transient in nature and easily treatable with aspirin or other pain relievers. Or they might report some degree of blurred vision, eye strain, or a feeling of light-headedness. Some patients notice increased irritability. However, these sensations pass quickly following the end of that day's phototherapy session, and are usually not experienced after the third or fourth day. Nonetheless they may cause patients to feel concerned about the treatment, and may diminish their enthusiasm for continuing with the program.

Even those who experience no adverse reactions might begin to doubt the value of the treatment. To a large extent, such negativism is hardly surprising, since depressed individuals tend to be pessimistic anyway. Or they may be concerned about the impact of the therapy on their lives, and the sessions will cut into their time at work or with the family.

On the third or fourth day of therapy, some of our patients experience a hypomanic episode during which their mood is abnormally high or they feel excessively stimulated. For most of these patients, this episode is followed by feelings of fatigue, which can reduce their enthusiasm for continuing with the program. Fortunately, after this episode, patients quickly return to a normal level of functioning.

During the maintenance phase, however, some patients may continue to feel hypomanic. If so we reduce the dosage of light until the patient feels more comfortable. Conversely, there are reports of some patients who actually feel more depressed during therapy with lights; perhaps these individuals suffer from "reverse SAD." In one case, a teenage boy whose condition grew worse under the lights was found to have a form of epilepsy that apparently affected his ability to respond to phototherapy.

One associated problem is that some patients using the lights at home tend to feel so much better than they did during their depressed periods that they feel they no longer need therapy. A few days after they quit, however, they may experience an emotional "crash," one that seems even more severe because of its contrast to the period of good feeling that preceded it. We try to emphasize to our patients that phototherapy is a *treatment*, not a cure, for SAD, and that lights must continue to be used throughout the winter.

Among the other concerns patients have is that they will not use the lights properly outside the clinical setting. We try to resolve this through careful counseling and by making ourselves available to answer any questions they might have.

Studies on the effects of phototherapy have found that the patient's ability to see is not affected following treatment. For some patients, however, the possibility that long-term use of the lights will cause eye damage is a matter for concern. While it may turn out that UV light may be an essential component of phototherapy, excessive amounts of UV rays are known to produce retinal damage and can lead to the development of cataracts. We take great care to explain to our patients that the UV radiation produced by phototherapy bulbs is kept to a minimum, and that only a few light sources, including the sun, lasers, and welding arcs, produce sufficient UV to pose a risk to the eyes. A study by the National Eye Institute found no evidence of physical damage to the eye after two weeks of exposure to bright light amounting to six hours a day. So far, at least, there have been no reports of eye damage caused by the use of phototherapy; we certainly have seen no evidence of it in our experience at Fair Oaks. The question is an important one, however. The use of antidepressant light therapy is a recent development, and continuing long-term studies are needed to provide conclusive evidence of its safety.

While we're on the subject, we must emphasize that phototherapy is not the medical equivalent of a trip to the tanning parlor. It is actually quite the opposite. Tanning lights generate high amounts of UV light in order to activate the skin-darkening process, which we'll explain in more detail in the next chapter. Tanners wear protective goggles to keep the light from entering their eyes. As we have seen, however, phototherapy requires patients to glance directly at the lights. Although getting a tan has its own degree of therapeutic value—especially if obtained while lounging on a tropical beach over a three-week period in February while sipping a frosty-cold drink—it is absolutely wrong to equate a tanning session with a phototherapy session.

One final concern about phototherapy: Some people who suffer from depression and who hear about the virtues of phototherapy may conclude that they can design a therapeutic strategy on their own. After all, they may think, I don't need to pay a doctor to tell me how to sit in front of a lamp. For those so inclined, we must emphasize that depression is a serious illness that requires the attention of medical professionals. You would not dream of performing surgery on yourself; likewise, you should not attempt to undertake this or any other form of therapy without first consulting a doctor.

In the next chapter we'll discuss medication and psychotherapy, the other key elements necessary for the complete treatment of SAD in many patients.

CHAPTER 7

OTHER TREATMENTS FOR SAD

Our enthusiasm for the use of phototherapy in treating Seasonal Affective Disorder is obvious. For our patients with depression who have tried just about everything else, a healthy dose of light added to their treatment regimen can be, literally, just what the doctor ordered. Other physicians have reported that in some cases, lights may be the only form of treatment necessary to produce improvement, especially for patients whose depression is relatively mind.

In most cases, however, phototherapy is just one element in the overall strategy for managing seasonal depression. The other legs of the "treatment triangle" are the judicious, carefully monitored use of antidepressant medications and a program of psychotherapy designed to address the needs of an individual patient.

At this point we should note again that, as a rule, the patients we see at Fair Oaks suffer from moderate to severe depression. Their histories usually show that they have been treated by a number of physicians and that they have been tried on a number of different medications before coming to us. Consequently, we are likely to take a different approach to the use of these therapies than if our patients were just beginning to seek treatment. The following discussion, however, is intended to give a general idea of the approach many psychiatrists might take in devising a therapeutic strategy for their patients with SAD.

Let's begin with an overview of the types of medications available. Published studies have reported that at least some SAD patients have found relief with each of these different classes of medications.

TRICYCLIC ANTIDEPRESSANTS

The revolution in treatment for depression began in the mid-1950s when a Swiss psychiatrist tested a chemical compound called imipramine. His intention was to compare imipramine to a related substance, chlorpromazine, which had been used successfully in the treatment of schizophrenia. Imipramine didn't help patients with that disorder, but it proved effective in cases of severe depression.

Chemically, imipramine possesses a distinctive structure: its atoms are assembled into three interlocking rings—a schematically truncated version of the Olympic logo. Because of this three-ring structure, imipramine and the other chemicals that resemble it are called *tricyclic antidepressants*, or TCAs. In the last three decades, a number of tricyclics have been introduced, each with its own niche in the armamentarium of medications. So effective are these chemicals that they are usually thought of as the "first line of treatment" for depression.

In addition to imipramine (sold under the brand name of Tofranil), the most commonly used TCAs and their brand names are:

amitriptyline (Elavil)
desipramine (Norpramin, Pertofrane)
doxepin (Sinequan)
nortriptyline (Aventyl, Pamelor)
protriptyline (Vivactil)
trimipramine (Surmontil)

Among the newly developed antidepressants—the so-called "second generation" antidepressants—are amoxapine (Asendin), fluoxetine (Prozac), maprotiline (Ludiomil) and trazodone (Desyrel). These antidepressants, while not technically considered TCAs, are similar in structure and effects.

Exactly how these medicines work is unclear. Physiologically speaking, depression arises due to some malfunction in the body systems responsible for producing and regulating two neurotransmitters, norepinephrine and serotonin, which are known to play a role in mood regulation. Some experts believe that depression occurs because the cells produce insufficient supplies of these chemicals. Others hold that the problems lies in the receptor sites—the "landing strips" where neurotransmitters connect the nerve cells. When these receptors become overly sensitive to the presence of neurotransmitters, depression can result. Tricyclic medications may serve to regulate secretion of neurotransmitters, or they may serve to reduce sensitivity in the receptor sites. In any case, they work, and they work dramatically.

One reason tricyclic antidepressants may work to treat SAD is that they also affect the body's circadian rhythms. Such action may help to normalize a disturbed rhythm, such as that of melatonin secretion. In addition, experiments have shown that unlike other psychoactive medications, antidepressants can help promote the body's ability to entrain circadian rhythms following a period of disruption. Thus, these medications may help to stabilize rhythms in patients with psychiatric disorders. As a rule, however, it takes ten days or more for medications to reach their full therapeutic efficacy, while with phototherapy, results may be seen as early as two days after treatment begins.

Because SAD is a relatively recent phenomenon, there have been few studies designed to compare the effectiveness of different types of treatments for the disorder. However, one team of researchers did conclude that the therapeutic effects of an hour of bright light a day were roughly equal to those seen following the use of imipramine (sold under the brand name

Tofranil). And of course the risk of side effects was much less for phototherapy than for treatment with medication.

Each TCA offers a slightly different combination of therapeutic benefits and drawbacks. Some treat just depression; others may also be effective in handling other associated psychiatric problems such as insomnia or anxiety. They all require a significant amount of time—up to six weeks—before they become fully effective. The dose must be carefully adjusted for each patient. And of course, every medication poses the risk of side effects. With TCAs, these can range from sedation to constipation, dizziness, or rapid pulse.

MONOAMINE OXIDASE (MAO) INHIBITORS

Like the TCAs, the MAO inhibitors used for depression are the descendants of a medication that had been used to treat a different illness entirely. In this case, the chemical is iproniazid and the disease it was used against was tuberculosis. TB patients given this substance seemed to become uncharacteristically cheerful. In the mid-1950s researchers began to investigate this unusual property of this chemical and its potential use in the treatment of depression. In so doing they created a new class of medications.

The MAO inhibitors derive their name from monoamine oxidase, an enzyme whose function is to break down neurotransmitters once they have penetrated a brain cell. Any medication that inhibits this activity will therefore serve to regulate the changes in mood that result from the presence of neurotransmitters. Unfortunately, an MAO inhibitor works not just in the brain but other cells throughout the body, resulting in the risk of such unwanted effects as dangerously increased blood pressure. Because of such drawbacks, many physicians became concerned about these medications and stopped prescribing them. Thus many patients who could have benefited from their therapeutic properties were unable to do so.

Further research, however, revealed that the increase in

blood pressure occurred when an MAO inhibitor was combined with other medications or foods, such as aged meats and cheese, that contained a substance known as tyramine, the so called "cheese reaction."

Thus in recent years MAO inhibitors have returned to favor as a useful method of treating depression. These medications are safe if the patient can reliably follow a list of foods and medications to avoid. Among the MAO inhibitors currently available are isocarboxacid (Marplan), phenelzine (Nardil), and tranylcypromine (Parnate). Because they have a different mechanism of action than tricyclics, MAO inhibitors may work for patients in whom TCAs prove ineffective. They are not usually considered to be the first choice, however; thus they are sometimes referred to as "second-line" medications. However, some researchers believe they may be particularly effective for atypical depression, and therefore may be appropriate for SAD.

OTHER OPTIONS: LITHIUM, ANTI-CONVULSANTS, AND BETA-BLOCKERS

The ability of lithium to stabilize mood swings was recognized as long as 1949; it took nearly twenty years, however, before this finding was applied to the treatment of mania and manic depression. As we have seen, people with manic depression experience periods of extreme mood elevation marked by high energy, euphoria, impulsivity, and impaired judgement. These periods alternate with plunges into lethargy, despair, and, all too frequently, suicidal thoughts or actions. For many people, lithium has literally been a lifesaver.

In some cases the use of lithium alone, or lithium in combination with a TCA, may not be producing the expected results. Lithium is known to slow down the functions of the thyroid gland. Thus some patients improve when given supplemental thyroid hormone to offset the slowing action of lithium. Lithium has also been shown to benefit some patients with PMS.

The anti-convulsants carbamazepine (Tegretol) and valproic

acid (Depakene) have been shown to be effective in manic depression patients not responsive to lithium. They may be particularly helpful in the "rapid-cyclers" or unstable mood disorders, having a positive effect on the limbic system.

Beta-blockers (such as propranolol and timolol) are named for their action in blocking the receptor sites that respond to adrenaline (epinephrine). They are not literally antidepressants, but have been used primarily to treat cardio-vascular disorders such as hypertension, arrhythmia, myocardial infarction (heart attacks), and angina.

Because the beta-blockers diminish symptoms associated with fright, stress, and hyperarousal (rapid heart beats, palpitations, and high blood pressure), they have been used to treat anxiety. Since melatonin is partially under the control of the beta receptor, beta-blockers have been considered in the treatment of SAD. Initial results are not impressive; however, more studies are needed before the efficacy—or lack of efficacy—of beta-blockers in SAD can be definitively established. In addition, beta-blockers must be used carefully since they themselves may actually cause depression.

However, one recent study is noteworthy. This study cites the case of a woman who suffered from pre-menstrual syndrome (PMS) only in the fall and winter. Use of phototherapy eliminated her symptoms. As an experiment, her doctors gave her an oral dose of melatonin, which, as predicted, reversed the beneficial effects of light. They then gave her doses of the beta-blockers propranolol and atenolol, medications that act to block the neural pathways responsible for triggering secretion of melatonin. With her melatonin thus suppressed by the beta-blocker, she again experienced relief from her PMS symptoms comparable to that she experienced during phototherapy. Other studies also find that atenolol given late in the afternoon can produce a dramatic impact on the pattern of melatonin secretion. Future research will help identify the role these medications may have in managing the onset and symptoms associated with SAD.

DETERMINING THE MEDICATION STRATEGY

We have briefly described the medications available for the treatment of depression in order to give you some idea of the choices confronting the physician. However there is more—much more—to the decision than merely selecting a medicine from the "shopping list" of available products and hoping that it works.

For one thing, unlike aspirin or cough syrups, antidepressants need time to take effect. Even at full strength, anywhere from ten days to three weeks must pass before real improvement is observed. But good medical practice demands that treatment begin with the lowest possible doses. Thus another three weeks may elapse while the physician adjusts the dosage to the level needed to produce the maximum effect. In many cases, this level is only found after the patient notices one or more adverse side effects, such as drowsiness or dry mouth. At that point the dosage is cut back and the response monitored for another few weeks. Eventually the regimen that produces the best results with the fewest adverse effects is found.

This approach works for about half of depressed patients. What about the other half? For them, the process takes longer. If one medication or a class of medications fails to work, the patient will be given a different product of the same class, or will be given a combination of medicines, or will be switched to a different therapeutic class entirely. More time must elapse while the response is monitored and the dosage adjusted. As long as six months may pass before the right medication (or combination) is found.

Of course, during this time, a depressed patient may begin to despair that any treatment will ever work and may drop out of treatment altogether. And of course, for a patient with SAD, six months is actually longer than it would take for the seasonal depression to lift on its own anyway. As spring approaches, a SAD patient may begin to feel better and may stop using medications altogether. For these reasons steps must be taken to reduce the guesswork involved.

We discussed some of these steps in previous chapters. One, of course, is to obtain a careful history of the problem and of the treatments used previously. Careful physical examination will determine whether some other organic or psychiatric illness is present. Sometimes too a patient must be referred for treatment at an alcohol- or drug-rehabilitation center to eliminate the effects of substance abuse or addiction.

Lab tests such as the thyrotropin-releasing hormone (TRH) test can be very helpful. This and other neuroendocrine tests will help determine whether there is some physical basis for the depression, and will help guide the choice of which medication to use. Conversely, consistently negative results on such tests may indicate that the patient will not be helped by antidepressants but may respond to psychotherapy alone.

Of course, if we suspect SAD, we will usually begin phototherapy immediately. However, if the patient also appears to be a candidate for antidepressant therapy, how do we determine which one to use? Since most of our patients are already using a first-line antidepressant, our first step is to check the patient's blood levels to see if the patient is receiving a therapeutic dose of the antidepressant. If a full therapeutic dose has not proven successful, then we will usually add either lithium or a thyroid hormone to the antidepressant. If this combination does not prove effective, then a second antidepressant—with a different mode of action—is usually tried. For some patients whose fatigue, drowsiness, and hypersomnia proves especially troublesome, a more stimulating antidepressant—such as desipramine (Norpramin) or tranylcypromine (Parnate)—may be more effective.

One way of predicting response is to give the patient a test dose of a certain medication and measure the amount that remains in the blood twenty-four hours later. Such data help determine the dosage that would be right for a patient, cutting down on the trial-and-error approach to prescribing.

We must also take into account the impact that a medication's side effects might have on a patient's lifestyle. For some people—

for example, an outpatient who teaches school—a medicine that produces drowsiness and a dry mouth would be unacceptable. In others—perhaps an inpatient who suffers from insomnia—the same side effect might actually be desirable.

Regardless of the approach chosen, we monitor the patient's reaction closely by drawing blood samples and determining the levels of the medication present. Such tests help us determine quickly and accurately whether the dosage we have chosen is working or whether it is merely posing the risk of unnecessary adverse effects.

One problem makes our work as physicians particularly difficult: the problem of compliance. It's a sad fact that, despite a physician's best efforts, regardless of the number of tests that are conducted, a segment of patients simply do not comply with their treatment program as prescribed. Either they take their medications at the wrong time or in the wrong amounts, or they fail to use them entirely. A percentage of patients who have been labeled "treatment resistant"—or those who do not benefit from therapy—are actually people who have simply failed to follow their treatment plan. And some SAD patients find the use of phototherapy to be inconvenient or unpleasant. These patients would rather take a pill than sit in front of the light box. Consequently we as physicians must be particularly vigilant to make sure our patients are following our instructions. In the hospital setting this is fairly easy to do; for outpatients, however, the problem is greater.

Nonetheless, despite the physician's enlightened choice of treatments, and despite careful monitoring, as many as fifteen percent of patients simply don't respond to the original prescribed medication. At that point we will decide whether to switch to another tricyclic, or an MAO inhibitor, or use some other combination. And for a certain number of patients, electroconvulsive therapy (ECT, or electroshock) may be called for.

Of course, treatment does not end with our signature on a prescription. We must continue to work with the patient to monitor progress. Followup testing will indicate the physiological response to medications, and will help us learn whether the patient is continuing to improve or is heading for a relapse. Our in-person conversations can help us determine how the patient is responding emotionally to treatment, and whether the life situations that may have triggered the depressive episode are improving. In cases of SAD, our first goal of course is to help the patient get through the dark months. However we must also stay in close touch over the spring and summer to watch for signs of hypomania, and must work together to anticipate the time when the days begin to grow shorter and a return to phototherapy will be needed.

Antidepressant medications are an invaluable resource in treating many forms of mental illness, and have revolutionized the management of depression. However, when used by themselves they are generally less effective for the patient with a clear-cut diagnosis of Seasonal Affective Disorder. These patients need the benefits that phototherapy can offer. And hard evidence is accumulating to suggest that antidepressants and light, when used in combination, produce more effect working together than either one does working alone. This combination is especially helpful for the 10 to 20 percent of patients who are not helped by phototherapy alone.

There is one other component to the treatment of SAD which can produce a number of solid, long-term benefits. That element is psychotherapy.

THE ROLE OF PSYCHOTHERAPY

Psychotherapeutic counseling in SAD is not aimed at relieving the symptoms of the disorder. Phototherapy and medications do that. Instead, psychotherapy—"talk therapy"—is effective when used to supplement other forms of treatment because it helps patients cope with the impact of the illness on virtally every facet of their lives. In a previous chapter we cited numerous example of how SAD can disrupt relationships among families and friends, and how the disorder can affect a person's ability to function creatively and effectively on the job. Psychotherapy helps patients to recognize the personal and social impact of seasonal depression, to confront and deal with their feelings, and to develop some practical ways of coping with their illness. A number of studies have established conclusively that in cases of severe depression, the use of certain kinds of psychotherapy in combination with medications is a more effective cure than medications alone.

We should perhaps note that the talk therapy we are dealing with here is not psychoanalysis, in which patients undergo years of soul-searching to get at the deep-rooted and deeply buried causes of their behavior. That approach isn't very useful for a patient with SAD, the cause of whose disorder is not an Oedipal struggle with parents but a malfunction in the body clock that responds to the light-dark cycle. Instead, psychotherapy for SAD (and other types of depression) is focused on the way patients think and act "in the here and now." Such therapy concentrates on acting to correct the present difficulty, not on gaining insights into the dim dark past. It helps patients adjust behavior to help them manage their lives on a day-to-day basis and is short-term, usually lasting for about six months or so.

If talk therapy of the here-and-now, in addition to medical treatment of their depression, is unsuccessful, other forms of therapy—including psychanalytically-based therapy—should be considered. Finding the right approach, and the right professional, requires time and effort.

TYPES OF PSYCHOTHERAPY

Individual therapy—one-to-one conversations with a professional—can be very important. Giving SAD patients the chance to focus on and express their feelings in a supportive, nonjudgmental environment can help uncover areas of real pain and suffering. Some patients feel an enormous sense of guilt because of the way they treated other members of their families during their depressed periods. The chance to express such feelings is an important step in learning positive ways to confront them and manage them.

Interpersonal therapy focuses on the disrupted relationships in a patient's life. Depression colors the way a person feels about and interacts with others; usually that color is black. Sometimes the symptoms of depression cause the disruption; at other times the disruptions trigger the depression. Often the conflict stems from the patient's role in life: One person might feel powerless when it comes to expressing her needs or desires to her husband; another might feel his wife will abandon him if he doesn't get a better job. While interpersonal therapy has only been in use for about a decade, it has already proved its usefulness in restoring shattered lives. By looking at depression within the patient's social setting, the therapist can spot the ways the illness impinges on the patient's life and can help identify the alternatives available to improve the situation.

Group therapy has particular advantages for certain SAD patients. Many times people are reluctant to accept advice from a physician; perhaps they feel doctors are out of touch with the realities that patients confront, or that they don't understand a particular need or feeling. Yet the same advice coming from a peer within the group setting can have tremendous impact. Hearing that another person has experienced the same emotion or dealt with the same problem can be an eye-opening experience. Patients can draw a great deal of support from one another as they open their hearts and reveal the difficulties they have experienced. Such group sessions are also a wonderful means for the exchange of practical tips on coping with the illness, such as how to use the lights properly or how to deal with the coming holiday season. Another advantage is that group sessions help reinforce other psychotherapeutic efforts. When patients hear the same remark made by both the physician and another SAD patient, they are more likely to trust the physician during future conversations.

Also, patients often develop their social skills within a group context. A patient who has withdrawn from social contact because of her disorder may be helped by phototherapy, but over the years may have become shy about initiating conversations with people she has not met. The encouragement and sympathy she receives from others in the group may help bolster her self-confidence and work to alleviate her shyness.

The use of *cognitive therapy* can help alter a patient's negative attitudes. The goal of cognitive therapy is to correct the faulty perception of the world by identifying false and distorted assumptions ("I'm a failure") and replacing them with a more balanced view. For example, a patient might say "I know I'll never get that promotion I really want." Repeated often enough, such an attitude makes the patient refuse even to apply for the desired position. Then, when the job is given to someone else, the patient moans, "See! I knew I wouldn't get it. I was right. I am a loser." In the process of cognitive therapy, however, the patient works closely with the therapist to learn to recognize how these self-defeating attitudes get translated into self-defeating behavior. Thus he or she comes to learn that the feeling of hopelessness is merely a symptom of the illness, not an inexorable condition. The next time a position opens up, the patient might hear himself say, "I know I won't get that job . . ." and automatically substitute another, more positive thought, such as ". . . unless I show the boss how good I'd be at it."

Family counseling, conducted in the presence of one or more members of the patient's family, helps spouses, children, and other relatives understand the nature of the patient's illness. Children may be particularly puzzled by their parents' yearly mood swings, and may feel that they are in some way to blame. Learning that SAD is caused by the changing seasons, and is not a personal reaction to them or to their behavior, can relieve guilt considerably. What's more, when family members come to understand the disorder and how the use of the light units can relieve symptoms, they are more willing to accept the treatment and to support their SAD-afflicted relative during the course of therapy. During a session, we as physicians are able to observe the way family members interact with one another. Hearing how problems are dealt with, or seeing the reactions of one person to the comments or behavior of another, can lead to a much greater understanding of the situation that confronts the patient and home. This in turn helps to make it easier for us to design and implement treatment.

Almost by definition, depression causes those with the illness to experience a negative view of the world. Depressed people are pessimistic, fatalistic, and feel hopeless about their situation. "I'm a failure," they'll say; "I'm no good; nobody loves me or ever will." Patients must deal with friends and family who cannot understand the basis for this negative attitude. Often their frustrated relatives will demand, "Why don't you just snap out of it?" Of course, if defeating SAD was just a question of "snapping out of it," many patients would have done so long ago.

In some cases, *marital therapy* may be needed to help repair the damage to a relationship that may have occurred during the patient's "down times." It is often the case that feelings of bitterness, sadness, or anger erupt during seasonal mood swings. The hurtful words exchanged during these times, or the patient's withdrawal from the mate, or the very instability of the relationship, can easily produce lasting scars. Unfortunately, the emotional and marital discord caused by SAD may even lead to divorce proceedings. Some patients will find that talking to a marital counselor can help restore the love and trust that were lost during the dark days.

SAD is particularly devastating to those patients who work. For many people, their feelings of worth and self-esteem are inextricably tied up with their ability to perform on the job. Thus *vocational counseling* can help some SAD patients recognize their strengths and their weaknesses, and can help identify jobs or careers that might be better suited to people with seasonal depression. Furthermore, a skilled vocational counselor may be able to suggest ways the patient can improve relationships with bosses and co-workers. Some SAD patients have been able to enlist the support of their employers during the phototherapeutic process. For example, a number have been able to set up lights in their offices or workspaces and use them in such a way as to avoid interfering with the everyday operation of the office. Some employers have been found to cooperate enthusiastically when they learn that use of the lights can improve their employee's ability to function, increases productivity, reduces absenteeism, and can help make it possible for a valuable worker to remain on the job. Such rare individuals are truly "enlightened."

One important aspect of counseling is often overlooked when it comes to managing SAD. As we have seen, the carbohydrate cravings that accompany bouts of depression can lead to a weight gain of 20 pounds or more. Often patients can lose that weight again in the spring. As time goes on, however, it becomes harder and harder to shed excess pounds. Many people experience feelings of shame or guilt associated with these changes in body weight. Thus *nutritional counseling* can help patients improve their diets, making it easier to take weight off and keep it off.

Regardless of the psychotherapeutic approach used, the process can take time and is not without its problems. Cost can be a factor, although many types of therapy are at least partly reimbursable under medical insurance plans. Another problem is the lack of commitment many patients feel toward such strategies. Again, this attitude may stem from their illness itself, which produces a pervasive sense of negativity and hopelessness. And the seasonal cycling of SAD creates a situation in which patients feel so good for half the year that they tend to believe they no longer need any kind of psychotherapeutic support. It's a strange phenomenon we have seen over and over in our SAD patients: The use of phototherapy, in combination with the other strategies, makes patients feel so much better that they forget exactly what it is that's causing their improvement. "I feel so much better; I think I'll skip the lights today," they might say, or, "I don't need to go to my group therapy session. I'm cured." Part of our jobs as physicians is to convince these patients, and remind them repeatedly, that it is their very participation in the therapeutic program that has brought them the improvement we both are seeking.

* * *

The purpose of this book has been to shed light on Seasonal Affective Disorder: to define it, to show how it affects the lives of people who suffer from it, and to outline the course of therapy. Future research will undoubtedly provide answers to the many questions that remain concerning the biological malfunctions that produce such a disorder and the tools needed to repair the damage.

The existence of SAD, and the realization that bright light is an extremely powerful therapeutic weapon, has made many medical professionals, ourselves among them, aware that a patient's complaint of feeling "under the weather" is much more than a mere cliché. It is a profoundly significant clue to the inner workings of our bodies and our minds.

CHAPTER 8

QUESTIONS AND ANSWERS

Q. *"Every winter you see articles in newspapers and reports on TV discussing people who get depressed when they don't get enough sunlight. What are they talking about?"*

A. Researchers are finding that we humans are attuned to our environment and are governed by natural cycles and rhythms to a much greater degree than we had previously suspected. These rhythms regulate a number of important body functions, including our moods.

Some body rhythms are regulated by exposure to sunlight over the course of a day. Both the amount and the timing of that exposure are important in keeping the different rhythms operating in harmony with one another.

We now know that some people are extraordinarily sensitive to the amount of light they receive. In the winter, as the days grow shorter, these people begin to feel and act differently. Their moods become more and more depressed, their energy wanes, and they suffer several other physical, mental, and emotional problems. The syndrome has been named Seasonal Affective Disorder, usually abbreviated to SAD. (In its medical sense "affect" means "mood.")

• • •

Q. *"When my husband learned I had been diagnosed as having seasonal depression, he said it sounded like the latest 'disease of the month.' Is he right? Is SAD just a fad?"*

A. Definitely not. Granted, some illnesses—hypoglycemia and "yuppie flu" for example—do seem to capture the public fancy for a while. These illnesses serve as convenient catch-all diagnoses for ailments that seem to have no other explanation, then fade from popularity as the next "hot contender" comes along.

Such is not the case with SAD. When the syndrome was first recognized in the early 1980s, research was undertaken to determine whether it was a truly distinct clinical entity. Within a short time SAD had been carefully defined and identified in hundreds of patients. So convincing was the evidence for SAD that only six short years elapsed before it was recognized as an "official" diagnosis by the medical community and included in the official list of true psychiatric disorders.

• • •

Q. *"In the summer I'm a lively, energetic, outgoing person. But every winter all I feel like doing is sleeping all day. I eat a lot of junky food, put on weight, and I turn grouchy and mean. My family thinks I would feel better if I would just go into hibernation for the rest of the season. Are they right—am I part bear?"*

A. What you are experiencing are the classic symptoms of SAD. People with this disorder often begin to feel a sense of dread when the leaves change color. They develop an overwhelming desire to sleep extra hours—as many as 12, 14, even 16 hours a day. Even with extra sleep, however, they awake feeling unrested and can barely drag themselves out of bed.

SAD patients also experience changes in their eating habits, usually in the form of uncontrollable cravings for sweet, starchy foods. Naturally, with all those extra carbohydrates, coupled with their decreased energy and activity, they tend to gain weight—sometimes as much as 50 pounds. A number of SAD patients own a separate "winter wardrobe" to accommodate their increasing bulk.

And of course the main hallmark of SAD is the depressed mood it inflicts on its victims. This depression can take the form of sadness, melancholy, and a withdrawal from friends and family.

Adding to the suffering caused by the disorder are other symptoms, such as decreased ability to concentrate, loss of libido, and increased physical complaints ranging from muscle aches to greater susceptibility to physical ailments. Naturally these problems can wreak havoc on an individual's family life, social relationships, and job performance.

• • •

Q. *"Who can get SAD? Is it contagious?"*
A. No, it is not contagious, but you may have inherited a tendency to develop the illness. Many SAD patients have relatives who suffer from psychiatric illnesses such as depression or alcoholism.

Estimates are that as many as five million Americans may have the disorder. SAD can strike anyone, but it affects three or four times as many women as men. Symptoms of SAD may resemble those of Premenstrual Syndrome and thus may not be recognized immediately.

SAD can start in childhood, but the average age at which people first notice symptoms is about 23. Many women have noticed that their illness began after they gave birth to a child. Because the disease cycles over the course of a year, many patients don't notice the pattern and thus seek help only after years have passed and the syndrome has grown progressively worse. A significant percentage of SAD patients have been previously treated for some kind of depression; some of these have been hospitalized at one time or another.

• • •

Q. *"How do doctors know that someone has SAD and not some other problem?"*
A. In recent years a careful definition of the disorder has been developed to help physicians recognize the condition in their patients. This definition distinguishes between seasonal depres-

sion and other types, including manic depressive illness, major depressive episode, borderline personality disorders, and so on.

The key to recognizing SAD, as its name suggests, is its persistent *seasonal* pattern: onset in fall/winter, remission in the spring; occurrence over a span of three years, and so on. Any seasonal stresses (holidays, unemployment) must be ruled out as factors.

• • •

Q. *"Do I have to just put up with this illness, or is there any kind of effective treatment or cure?"*

A. Treatment for SAD involves the use of precisely controlled and administered bright light. While other types of therapy—medications and psychotherapy—can help relieve symptoms of depression, most patients with SAD will only experience maximum benefit through exposure to light.

The effectiveness of phototherapy is quite dramatic. Results can be seen usually within one to four days, compared to the weeks or months needed for medications to take effect. The lights continue to relieve depression throughout the winter. In the spring, when the amount of sunlight increases, patients can stop using the lights. Phototherapy is not a cure, however. The lights must be used each year when depression recurs.

• • •

Q. *"Will I have to sit in front of lights all day? Will the lights hurt my eyes or cause skin cancer?"*

A. Most patients seem to benefit from phototherapy that lasts about an hour a day, usually in the morning or early afternoon. Patients look at the lights only for about ten seconds out of every minute; the rest of the time they may read or watch TV.

The lights are about as bright as sunlight seen from a window on a cloudless spring day and they do emit some ultraviolet light. Phototherapy bulbs are designed to replicate the spectrum of sunlight. The amount of UV is very small, however, and in nearly a decade of experience there has been no report of any eye damage to a patient undergoing phototherapy. Some patients do report temporary disturbances—blurry vision, minor headaches—which vanish soon after the therapy session has ended.

The most common side effect of light treatment is overstimulation. Should that occur, the solution is to reduce the dosage and administer phototherapy early enough in the day that any such overstimulation will not interfere with sleep.

• • •

Q. *"My doctor told me I should take walks on winter mornings, or go skiing as often as possible. But he said I shouldn't wear sunglasses or glasses with tinted lenses. How come?"*
A. There are several reasons. Getting outside during the day helps increase your exposure to sunlight and can thus supplement the benefits gained from phototherapy. Also, exercise, activity, and social stimulation are important to everyone's state of health, and can be of special value to patients with SAD. Skiing is particularly good because sunlight reflects off of snow.

The effects of phototherapy are transmitted through the eyes, and not through the skin. Wearing sunglasses would block out the light and thus reduce its therapeutic properties. (Of course you should never look directly at the sun for any reason.)

One other caution: phototherapy is not the equivalent of a trip to the tanning parlor. Tanning lamps generate high amounts of ultraviolet light, and tanners *must* wear sunglasses to protect their eyes from potential damage.

• • •

Q. *"Why do I need a doctor to treat this problem? I've read about SAD, I know about the light treatment. Why can't I just get a kit from the hardware store and build my own phototherapy unit?"*
A. SAD is a serious psychiatric illness. Like other illnesses it requires medical attention. A skilled physician can recognize the signs and symptoms, assess their degree of severity, and recommend appropriate treatment.

You would never perform surgery on yourself; likewise you should never self-diagnose and treat other ailments. You may misinterpret what you have read or misunderstand your symptoms. You may be suffering from a completely different type of illness, one that might actually worsen with phototherapy. And many patients with SAD require the supplemental use of antidepressant medications, which can only be supplied by professionals.

Phototherapy is no different from any other medicine. It should be used only under the supervision of a qualified physician.

• • •

Q. *"I've had SAD for years but I didn't know it. I didn't recognize the pattern—feeling blue every winter, quarreling with my husband and family, having difficulty at work—until last year, when my doctor diagnosed the problem. Phototherapy has really worked for me. I feel fifty times better, my career is really taking off. But I'm still having trouble with my family, and my marriage seems pretty shaky. How come?"*

A. Treatment for depression—seasonal or otherwise—is a complex affair. While phototherapy for SAD can bring about nearly instant improvement in mood, repairing the damage depression can cause to the patient's relationships with family, friends, and co-workers can take time. The anger, bitterness, and sense of withdrawal suffered during the "down times" can create scars that may require years to heal. And many SAD patients feel enormous guilt for the burden they have placed on their loved ones, who have also been forced to cope with the consequences of the illness.

Fortunately, a number of supportive therapies, ranging from family and group therapy to marital counseling, exist which can help patients mend the tattered fabric of their lives.

BIBLIOGRAPHY

Anonymous. The cruelest months. McLean Review (McLean Hospital, Belmont MA); Summer 1987:18-24.

Anonymous. Light therapy research discussed at Brookside depression symposium. Grand Rounds (Brookside Hospital publication), Dec 1986:1-3.

Anonymous. Research at PIA facility sheds new light on "winter blues." Network (NME newsletter), Feb 1987;17(2):8.

Anonymous. Solar power. United Airways Magazine, Sept 1986:48-50.

American Psychiatric Association: *Diagnostic and Statistical Manual of Mental Disorders, Third Edition, Revised.* Washington, DC: American Psychiatric Association, 1987.

Arato M, Rihmer Z, Szadoczky E. Seasonal influence on the dexamethasone suppression test results in unipolar depression (letter). Archives of General Psychiatry, Aug 1986;43:813.

Barley BG. New cures for depression. New Woman, Dec 1986:76-82.

Beck-Friis J, Borg G, Mellgren T et al. Nocturnal serum melatonin levels following evening bright light exposure. Clinical Neuropharmacology 1986;9(supp 4):184-186.

Beck-Friis J, Kjellman BF, Aperia B et al. Serum melatonin in relation to clinical variables in patients with major depressive disorder and a hypothesis of a low melatonin syndrome. Acta Psychiatr Scand 1985;71:319-330.

Bick, PA. Season major affective disorder. American Journal of Psychiatry Jan 1986;143:90-91.

Boyce P, Parker G. Seasonal Affective Disorder in the southern hemisphere. American Journal of Psychiatry, Jan 1988;145(1): 96-99.

Boyles, P. New light on winter darkness. Yankee, Feb 88:107ff.

Bramley FM. *Color: From Rainbows to Lasers.* New York: Thomas Y. Crowell Co., 1978.

Brewerton TD, Gwirtsman HE. Season dexamethasone suppression test results. Archives of General Psychiatry, Oct 1987;44:920-921.

Brower M. If winter's gloom gives you the blues, Norman Rosenthal may be able to lighten your mood. People Magazine, Jan 11 1988:115-116.

Costigan K: Cabin fever. Forbes, May 20 1985:234-238.

Daan S, Lewy AJ. Scheduled exposure to daylight: a potential strategy to reduce "jet lag" following transmeridian flight. Psychopharmacology Bulletin, 1984;20(3):566-568.

DeMet E, Chicz-DeMet A. Effects of psychoactive drugs on circadian rhythms. Psychiatric Annals, Oct 10, 1987:17:683-688.

The Diagram Group. *The Brain: A User's Manual.* New York: Berkley Books, 1982.

Docherty, J. Clinical assessment of Seasonal Affective Disorder. Summary of data presented at annual meeting of the APA, May 1987. (Unpublished)

Dullea G. Shedding light on dark-day blues. New York Times, Dec 19 1985:C1.

Evans C. At South Pole, sick bay is a one-man operation. New York Times, Apr 4, 1988.

Friend T: Blame dark days for winter blues. USA Today, 21 Dec 1987:1D.

Gadsby P: What light has to do with winter blues. Good Housekeeping, Feb 1985.

Garfield E. Chronobiology: an internal clock for all seasons. Part

2. Current research on Seasonal Affective Disorder and phototherapy. Current Comments; Jan 11 1988:3-9.

Garvey MJ, Wesner R, Godes M. Comparison of seasonal and nonseasonal affective disorders. American Journal of Psychiatry, Jan 1988;145(1):100-102.

Gever J: Brightening up the winter blues. Business NH, Dec 1986:69-71.

Goslin J: Brookside tests new drug for insomnia. The Telegraph, Jan 3 1988:F9.

Gwynne P: Banishing wintertime blues. Woman's Day, Mar 4 1986:24.

Hansen S. Treatment of seasonal affective disorder with light. Wisconsin Medical Journal, Feb 1987;86:9-10.

Hansen T, Bratlid T, Lingjaerde O et al. Midwinter insomnia in the subarctic region: evening levels of serum melatonin and cortisol before and after treatment with bright artificial light, Acta Psychiatr Scand 1987;75:428-434.

Hellekson CJ, Kline JA, Rosenthal NE. Phototherapy for Seasonal Affective Disorder in Alaska. American Journal of Psychiatry 1986;143:1035-1037.

Hole John W. Jr. *Human Anatomy and Physiology.* Dubuque, Iowa: Wm C. Brown Co., 1981.

Jacobsen FM, Rosenthal NE. Seasonal affective disorder and the use of light as an antidepressant. Directions in Psychiatry. U S Govt Printing Office, Dept HHS.

Jacobsen FM, Wehr TA, Sack DA et al: Seasonal affective disorder: a review of the syndrome and its public health implications. American Journal of Public Health, Jan 1987;77(1):57-60.

Jacobsen FM, Wehr TA, Skwerer RA et al. Morning- versus midday-phototherapy of Seasonal Affective Disorder. October 1986 (unpublished).

James SP, Wehr TA, Sack DA et al. The desamethasone suppression test in Seasonal Affective Disorder. Comprehensive Psychiatry, May/June 1986:27(3):224-226.

James SP, Wehr TA, Sack DA et al. Treatment of Seasonal Affective Disorder with evening light. Unpublished manuscript accepted by British Journal of Psychiatry, Feb 1985.

Joseph-Vanderpool JR, Rosenthal NE. Phototherapy for Seasonal Affective Disorder. Drug therapy, Jan 1988:57-64.

Kales A, Kales J: Evaluation and Treatment of Insomnia. New York: Oxford University Press, 1984.

Kasper S, Rogers S, Yancey A et al. Psychological effects of light therapy in normals. Unpublished ms, July 1987.

Kripke DF. Therapeutic effects of bright light in depressed patients. Annals New York Academy of Sciences 1984;453: 270-281.

Kripke DF. Treating depression with light: an interview with Daniel Kripke, MD. Currents, May, 1985;5-8.

Kripke DF, Risch SC, Janowsky D. Bright white light alleviates depression. Psychiatry Research 1983:10:105-112.

Kripke DF, Risch SC, Janowsky DS. Lighting up depression. Psychopharmacology Bulletin, 1983;19(3):526-530.

Lamola AA. A history of organizations interested in the biological effects of light. Annals New York Academy of Sciences 1984;453:121-122.

Levin EM. The Penetrating Beam, Reflections on Light. New York: Richards Rosen Press, Inc., 1978.

Lewy AJ, Kern HA, Rosenthal NE et al. Bright artificial light treatment of a manic-depressive patient with a seasonal mood cycle. American Journal of Psychiatry, Nov 1982;139(11):1496-1498.

Lewy AJ, Sack RL. Melatonin physiology and light therapy. Clinical Neuropharmacology 1986;9(suppl 4):196-198.

Lewy AJ, Sack RL, Fredrickson RH et al. The use of bright light in the treatment of chronobiologic sleep and mood disorders: the phase-response curve. Psychopharmacology Bulletin 1983;19(3):523-525.

Lewy AJ, Sack RL, Miller LS et al. Antidepressant and circadian phase-shifting effects of light. Science, Jan 16 1987;235:352-354.

Lewy AJ, Sack RA, Singer CM. Assessment and treatment of chronobiologic disorders using plasma melatonin levels and bright light exposure: the clock-gate model and the phase response curve. Psychopharmacology Bulletin, 1984;20(3):561-565.

Lewy AJ, Sack RL, Singer CM. Immediate and delayed effects

of bright light on human melatonin production: shifting "dawn" and "dusk" shifts the dim light melatonin onset (DLMO). Annals New York Academy of Sciences 1984;453:253-259.

Lewy AJ, Sack RL, Singer CM. Treating phase typed chronobiologic sleep and mood disorders using appropriately timed bright artificial light. Psychopharmacology Bulletin 1985;21 (3):368-372.

Lewy AJ, Siever LJ, Uhde TW et al. Clonidine reduces plasma melatonin levels. Journal of Pharmaceutical Pharmacology 1986;38:555-556.

Lewy AJ, Wehr TA, Goodwin FK et al. Light suppresses melatonin secretion in humans. Science, Dec 12 1980; 210: 1267-1268.

Lewy AJ, Wehr TA, Goodwin FK et al. Manic-depressive patients may be supersensitive to light. Lancet, Feb 14 1981:383-384.

Lewy AJ, Wehr TA, Rosenthal NE et al. Melatonin secretion as a neurobiological "marker" and effects of light in humans. Psychopharmacology Bulletin 1982;18(4):127-129.

Lincoln G. Melatonin as a seasonal time-cue: a commercial story. Nature, April 1983(?):775.

Lingjaerde O, Bratlid T, Hansen T et al. Seasonal Affective Disorder and midwinter insomnia in the far north: studies on two related chronobiological disorders in Norway. Clinical Neuropharmacology, 1986;9(suppl 4):187-189.

Maas JB, Jayson JK, Kleiber DA. Effects of spectral differences in illumination on fatigue. Journal of Applied Psychology, 1974;59(4):524-526.

Milbouer S: Light energizes victims of SAD. The Telegraph, Nashua, NH. Dec. 1986.

Milbouer S: Research may lighten 'SAD'ness. The Telegraph, Nashua, NH. Dec. 1986.

Moore RY, Card JP. Visual pathways and the entrainment of circadian rhythms. Annals New York Academy of Sciences 1984;453:123-133.

Morris R. Light. New York: The Bobbs-Merrill Co., 1979.

Mueller PS, Allen NG. Diagnosis and treatment of severe

light-sensitive seasonal energy syndrome (SES) and its relationship to melatonin anabolism. Psychiatry Letter (Fair Oaks Hospital Newsletter), Sept 1984;2(9):1-6.

Mueller PS, Davies RK. Seasonal Affective Disorders: seasonal energy syndrome? (Letter; reply by Rosenthal NE). Archives of General Psychiatry, Feb 1986;43:188-189.

Napoli M: Shedding light on the winter blahs. Family Circle, Feb 2 1988:24.

National Geographic Society: The Incredible Machine. Washington DC: National Geographic Society, 1986.

Neer RM, Davis TRA, Walcott A et al. Stimulation by artificial lighting of calcium absorption in elderly human subjects. Nature 222:255-257.

New York State Psychiatric Institute. 10,000 lux light therapy enhances SAD treatment effect. (Press release).

Parry BL, Rosenthal NE, Tamarkin L et al. Treatment of a patient with seasonal premenstrual syndrome. American Journal of Psychiatry 1987;144:762-766.

Ponte L: Staying happy in cold, dark winter. Reader's Digest, Jan 1984:86-89.

Potkin SG, Zetin M, Stamenkovic V et al. Seasonal affective disorder: prevalence varies with latitude and climate. Clinical Neuropharmacology, 1986;9(suppl 4):181-183.

Reader's Digest. ABC's of the Human Body: A Family Answer Book. Pleasantville, New York: The Reader's Digest Association, Inc., 1987.

Rensberger Boyce: Spring fever not imaginary, study finds. Washington Post, March 11, 1985, A5.

Rosenthal NE, Light as a treatment for seasonal depression: an interview with Norman Rosenthal, MD. Currents 5:5, May 1986.

Rosenthal NE, Carpenter CJ, James SP et al. Seasonal Affective Disorder in children and adolescents. American Journal of Psychiatry 1986;143:356-358.

Rosenthal NE, Lewy AJ, Wehr TA et al. Seasonal cycling in a bipolar patient. Psychiatry Research, 1983;8:25-31.

Rosenthal NE, Sack DA, Carpenter CJ et al. Antidepressant

effects of light in Seasonal Affective Disorder. American Journal of Psychiatry 1985; 142:163-170.

Rosenthal NE, Sack DA, Gillin JC et al. Seasonal Affective Disorder: a description of the syndrome and preliminary findings with light therapy. Archives of General Psychiatry, Jan 1984;41:72-80.

Rosenthal NE, Sack DA, Jacobsen FM et al. Consensus and controversy in Seasonal Affective Disorder and phototherapy. Abstract presented at the IVth World Congress of Biological Psychiatry, Philadelphia, Sept 1985.

Rosenthal NE, Sack DA, Jacobsen FM et al. The role of melatonin in Seasonal Affective Disorder (SAD) and phototherapy. Presented at the First International Congress on Melatonin in Humans, Vienna, Nov 1985.

Rosenthal NE, Sack DA, Jacobsen FM et al. Seasonal Affective Disorder and light: past, present and future. Clinical Neuropharmacology 1986;9(suppl 4):193-195.

Rosenthal NE, Sack DA, James SP et al. Seasonal Affective Disorder and phototherapy. Presented at New York Academy of Sciences, Nov 1984.

Rosenthal NE, Wehr TA. Seasonal Affective Disorders. Psychiatric Annals, Oct 1987;17(10):671-674.

Rossotti H. *Colour: Why the World Isn't Grey.* Princeton, New Jersey: Princeton University Press, 1983.

Rovner S. Children's moods and the light of day. Washington Post, Sept 11 1985.

Roy-Byrne PP, Rubinow DR, Hoban MC et al. Premenstrual changes: a comparison of five populations. Psychiatry Research, 1986;17:77-85.

Sherer MA, Weingartner H, James SP et al. Effects of melatonin on performance testing in patients with Seasonal Affective Disorder. Neuroscience Letters, 1985;58:277-282.

Stewart JW: Importance of timing and duration of phototherapy (letter; reply by Wehr, Sack, and Rosenthal). Archives of General Psychiatry, Oct 1987;44:921-923.

Stonehouse B, Brotherhood J, Ridley R. *The Way Your Body Works*. New York: Crown Publishers, Inc., 1974.

Thase M. Defining and treating Seasonal Affective Disorder. (Interview). Psychiatric Annals, Dec 12 1986;16:733-737.

Thompson C. Seasonal Affective Disorder and phototherapy: experience in Britain. Clinical Neuropharmacology, 1986;9(suppl 4):190-192.

Toufexis A. Dark days, darker spirits. Time, Jan 11 1988:66.

Verity E. *Color Observed*. New York: Van Nostrand Reinhold Co., 1980.

Wehr TA, Jacobsen FM, Sack DA et al. Phototherapy of Seasonal Affective Disorder. Archives of General Psychiatry 1986;43: 870-875.

Wehr TA, Sack DA, Rosenthal NE. Antidepressant effects of sleep deprivation and phototherapy. Acta Psyciat Belg 1985;85: 593-602.

Wehr TA, Skwerer RG, Jacobsen FM et al. Eye versus skin phototherapy of Seasonal Affective Disorder. American Journal of Psychiatry 1987;144:753-757.

Wehr TA, Wirz-Justice A, Goodwin FK et al. Phase advance of the circadian sleep-wake cycle as an antidepressant. Science, Nov 9 1979;206:710-713.

Wehr TA, Wirz-Justice A, Goodwin FK. Biological rhythm disturbances in affective illness. Biological Psychiatry Today, 1979:303-306.

Welch, B: Fever, disorder discussed (letter). The Telegraph, Mar 9 1987:16.

Wever RA. Use of light to treat jet lag: differential effects of normal and bright artificial light on human circadian rhythms. Annals New York Academy of Sciences, 1984;453:282-304.

Wirz-Justice A. Light therapy for depression: present status, problems, and perspectives. Psychopathology, 1986:19(suppl 2):136-141.

Wirz-Justice A, Arendt J. Diurnal, menstrual cycle, and seasonal indole rhythms in man and their modification in affective disorders. Biological Psychiatry Today, 1979:294-302.

Wirz-Justice A, Bucheli C, Schmid AC et al. A dose relationship in bright white light treatment of seasonal depression (letter). American Journal of Psychiatry, July 1986; 143(7):932-933.

Wirz-Justice A, Bucheli C, Graw P et al. Light treatment of Seasonal Affective Disorder in Switzerland. Acta Psychiatr Scand 1986;74:193-204.

Wirz-Justice A, Richter R. Seasonality in biochemical determinations: a source of variance and a clue to the temporal incidence of affective illness. Psychiatry Research, 1979;1:53-60.

Wirz-Justice A, Schmid AC, Graw P et al. Dose relationships of morning bright white light in Seasonal Affective Disorders (SAD). Experientia 1987;43:574-576.

Wurtman RJ. The effects of light on the human body. Scientific American, July, 1975.

Yerevanian BI, Anderson JL, Grota LJ et al. Effects of bright incandescent light on seasonal and nonseasonal major depressive disorder. Psychiatry Research 1986;18:355-364.

Zung WWK, Green RL. Seasonal variation of suicide and depression. Archives of General Psychiatry, Jan 1974;30:89-91.

INDEX

Other Books Available

The Good News About Depression, by Mark S. Gold, M.D.
The Good News About Panic, Anxiety and Phobias, by Mark S. Gold, M.D.
Sixty Ways to Make Stress Work For You, by Andrew E. Slaby, M.D., Ph.D., M.P.H.
Guide To The New Medicines Of The Mind, by Irl Extein, M.D., Larry S. Kirstein, M.D., and Peter Herridge, M.D.
The Facts About Drugs and Alcohol, 3rd edition, by Mark S. Gold, M.D.
Get Smart About Weight Control, by Phillip M. Sinaikin, M.D.
High Times/Low Times: The Many Faces of Adolescent Depression, by John E. Meeks, M.D.
On the Edge: The Love/Hate World of the Borderline Personality, by Neil D. Price, M.D.
Overcoming Insomnia, by Donald R. Sweeney, M.D., Ph.D.
Light Up Your Blues: Understanding and Overcoming Seasonal Affective Disorders, by Robert N. Moreines, M.D.
A Parent's Guide to Common and Uncommon School Problems, by David A. Gross, M.D. and Irl L. Extein, M.D.
Psychiatric Skeletons: Tracing the Legacy of Mental Illness In the Family, by Steven D. Targum, M.D.
Life On A Roller Coaster: Coping With the Ups and Downs of Mood Disorders, by Ekkehard Othmer, M.D., Ph.D., and Sieglinde C. Othmer, Ph.D.
A Consumer's Guide to Psychiatric Diagnosis, by Mark A. Gould, M.D.
Aftershock, by Andrew E. Slaby, M.D., Ph.D., M.P.H.
Kids Out of Control, by Alan M. Cohen, M.D.
A Parent's Guide To Teens and Cults, by Larry E. Dumont, M.D. and Richard I. Altesman, M.D.
The Family Contract, by Howard I. Leftin, M.D.
Family Addictions, A Guide For Surviving Alcohol and Drug Abuse, by Charles R. Norris, Jr., M.D.
Kids On the Brink: Understanding the Teen Suicide Epidemic, by David B. Bergman, M.D.
Codependency, Sexuality and Depression, by William E. Thornton, M.D.
When Self-Help Isn't Enough: Overcoming Addiction and Psychiatric Disorders, by A. Scott Winter, M.D.
No More Secrets, No More Shame: Understanding Sexual Abuse and Psychiatric Disorders, by David A. Sack, M.D.
Living with Pain by William S. Makarowski, M.D.
Living with Head Injury: A Guide for Families, by Richard C. Senelick, M.D., and Cathy E. Ryan
Kids Who Do/Kids Who Don't: A Parent's Guide To Teens and Drugs, by Lorraine Henricks, M.D.
Caught In the Crossfire: The Impact of Divorce on Young People, by Lorraine Henricks, M.D.
Teens At Risk, by Kevin Leehey, M.D.
Sit Down and Pay Attention, by Ronald Goldberg, M.D.
Save the Males, by Kenneth Wetcher, M.D., Art Barker, M.A., and F. Rex McCaughtry, M.S.W.

ABOUT THE AUTHORS

Robert N. Moreines, M.D. Director, Inpatient Services and Director of Education and Training at Fair Oaks Hospital. Dr. Moreines received his BA from Harvard University, and his M.D. from Michigan State. Dr. Moreines served as Chief Resident at Columbia. Dr. Moreines has authored book chapters on psychiatric diagnoses, maximizing efficacy of antidepressant medications, and treatment of schizophrenia.

Patricia L. McGuire, M.D. Before joining Fair Oaks Hospital, Dr. McGuire was an Instructor and then Assistant Professor, Department of Psychiatry and Human Behavior, Division of Biology and Medicine, Brown University. After graduating from Brown, Dr. McGuire completed medical school and her internship at Wayne State, and her psychiatric residency at Johns Hopkins Medical School. Following her residency, she was a Clinical Fellow in Psychiatry, Harvard Medical School, specializing in Consultation-Liaison Psychiatry.